The Pre-Dental Guide

The Pre-Dental Guide

a guide for successfully getting into dental school

Joseph S. Kim, DDS

Writers Club Press
San Jose New York Lincoln Shanghai

The Pre-Dental Guide
a guide for successfully getting into dental school

Writers Club Press
an imprint of iUniverse.com, Inc.

For information address:
iUniverse.com, Inc.
5220 S 16th, Ste. 200
Lincoln, NE 68512
www.iuniverse.com

ISBN: 0-595-19447-8

Printed in the United States of America

To Sara and Solomon…my inspiration and my joy.

Contents

Introduction

Congratulations on making the decision to enter the prestigious and exciting field of dentistry! You will soon join more than 160,000 dentists that are currently practicing in the United States alone. Of course, there is one minor obstacle in your way: getting into dental school. For many, the entire prospect of evaluating, choosing, and applying to a dental program is rather daunting.

The purpose of this book is to provide pre-dental students with pertinent information about the various factors to consider when choosing and applying to dental school. Also, the major elements of the Dental Admission Test, and advice on how to take it, will be looked at in some detail. In addition, this book makes recommendations regarding the pre-dental resources which are currently on the market.

As a former pre-dental student, test instructor, and dental student, I have tried to present this information in a straightforward and useful manner. I remember my own experience applying to dental school, and the lack of meaningful guidance that was available. Few pre-professional advisors, and even fewer books can satisfy the multitude of questions and concerns floating in the mind of a pre-dental student. Through this book, I have made every effort to ease your fears and concerns by anticipating and addressing those matters which are of importance to pre-dental students.

After reading this book, it is my sincere hope that you will gain the confidence and skills necessary to successfully enter the dental school of your choice. It will be a milestone in your life, as it is in mine, that you will not regret. Again, welcome to dentistry!

Joseph S. Kim, DDS

I.

So, you want to be a dentist?

1. Facts and Figures

"Dentists diagnose, prevent, and treat problems of the teeth and tissues of the mouth. They remove decay, fill cavities, examine x-rays, place protective plastic sealants on children's teeth, straighten teeth, and repair fractured teeth. They also perform corrective surgery of the gums and supporting bones to treat gum diseases. Dentists extract teeth and make molds and measurements for dentures to replace missing teeth. Dentists provide instruction in diet, brushing, flossing, the use of fluorides, and other aspects of dental care, as well. They also administer anesthetics and write prescriptions for antibiotics and other medications." [1]

There are many reasons for becoming a dentist. Some of these include having a member of your family in the profession, wanting some assurance of a six figure income, and the desire to have a more relaxed lifestyle than other professional occupations. Whatever your motivations and reasons may be, you've made the right choice.

---

[1] Cosca, Theresa, *Bureau of Labor Statistics*, Last modified: February 24, 1999 *URL: http://stats/bls.gov/oco/ocos072.htm*

Dentistry is a field that demands not only the skills and attention to details of an artist, but the scrutiny and acumen of a scientist. Dentistry is constantly changing with current advances in material science, medicine, pharmacology, and high tech advances. Dentistry will put you in contact with people who will appreciate your services, professional colleagues who will respect your expertise, and employees who will value your leadership. In a nutshell, the modern day dentist is excellent in the areas of esthetics, medicine, technology, and people skills.

Students who opt to pursue dentistry due, in part or in whole, to having some member of their family in the field may have a slight, but significant advantage over others when it comes to clinical performance in dental school. However, whether or not they take this advantage is up to them. While others may have only the vaguest ideas as to what real life dentistry entails, these students have a readily available opportunity to observe, help, and understand the concepts that are used daily in the profession. Also, they often have access to dental literature and books, as well as to the expertise of the family member. They have the opportunity to understand and utilize, in a limited fashion, the tools of the trade. Being in this boat, although arbitrary, is very good.

The opportunity to earn money can most certainly be found in this field. It is just a matter of finding the proper equilibrium of education and work versus income that will determine the final numbers. According to the American Dental Association, the average net income of general practice dentists in 1995 was $124,960. For those who were in a specialty practice, the average net income was $196,670. Also, recent wage surveys have demonstrated that the average dentist earns over $80 per hour compared with just over $70 per hour for physicians. It is important to note that these numbers reflect average incomes, with some earning more, and some earning less. Those who are just beginning their careers will probably have lower incomes, while those who have become established will earn higher amounts due to experience, speed, and a grasp of technical, diagnostic, and financial knowledge.

Dentistry is a comfortable field that will most likely always remain within the top ten income averages in the United States.

Some of the reasons for the average pay gap between general practitioners and specialists include overhead, expertise, and the higher fees that specialists command for similar if not the same procedures. The business overhead of the specialist if often lower than that of a general dentist. Specialists need only stock items, such as equipment and materials, that pertain to their particular field. Also, they have a lesser need to promote their services to the public. Rather, they usually make their presence known to local general dentists who ultimately refer patients who present with a situation beyond the scope and expertise of the general dentist, or who are difficult to manage. These "difficult" patients include those who are medically and systemically compromised, patients who are mentally or emotionally handicapped or otherwise unstable, and patients who are just difficult to work with.

Expertise in a particular field can generally be equated with higher education. With few exceptions, a specialist can be expected to be more knowledgeable and proficient with those modalities that are within their particular field. Also, increased familiarity with procedures and materials will usually be associated with assistants and other dental auxiliaries of the specialist. It is only logical to conclude that an assistant who participates in a focused area of dentistry will be more efficient and aware of their roles in the overall management of a limited category of patients.

Those who wish to enter dentistry to suit their particular lifestyle will be especially rewarded. Dentistry is best described as flexible. Recent surveys have found that the average dentist works 37.0 hours per week. And although this "flexibility" is not evident during the first few years of dental school as well as the first few years of practice, the choice is always there. Because this field differs from medicine in that most dentists will become general dentists (currently 79% according to the ADA), the type of competition that exists amongst classmates is entirely different from that of their medical school counterparts. Very few students fail due to poor grades, or lack of skill. Rather, it is usually due to lack of interest in the field, or other extenuating circumstances that will keep a student from completing his or her dental education. After dental school, the stresses of paying off educational loans, and the looming prospect of taking on even more debt to start a practice will, in many cases, translate into longer hours at work. However, it is but a short distance from this scenario to the more common caricature of the golfing dentist who works no more than four days a week. If the lifestyle is what brought you dentistry, you will have to pay your dues, but in the end it will have been worth it.

Specialties

One area that is probably the last thing on the minds of most pre-dental students is that of specialty dentistry. This should not be the case. When selecting a potential dental school, and when deciding the level of performance that will have to be achieved while in that school, having an idea in mind about whether or not you will specialize will be a tremendous asset. Currently, there are nine specialties recognized by the American Dental Association. These specialty fields are Dental Public Health, Endodontics, Oral and Maxillofacial Pathology, Oral and Maxillofacial Radiology, Oral and Maxillofacial Surgery, Orthodontics and Dentofacial Orthopedics, Pediatric Dentistry, Periodontics, and Prosthodontics. Of these, Orthodontics and Oral and Maxillofacial Surgery are the most popular, and thus, the most competitive specialty fields.

Dental Public Health deals with issues on a macroscopic scale. That is, it tries to solve the bigger problem rather than meet each individual's specific needs. For example, the introduction and scientific study of fluoride in community water was to a large degree the work of public health dentists. Identification of epidemic situations, advice to local, state, and federal governments, public service announcements, and scientific inquiry into trends and current states of dental and oral health are but a few of the wide range of issues and concerns addressed by public health dentists. In general, these dentists are experts in the area of epidemiology. You will find a large number of public health dentists working for the government on the local, state, and federal levels, as well as employed by all dental schools as educators and researchers. Today, the studies and strategies employed by communities and local governments to diminish dental disease are in the domain of Dental Public Health. Public health dentists can earn a Masters in Public Health (MPH), a Doctorate in Public Health (DrPH), or a Doctor of Philosophy (PhD) degree. The Masters program usually receives a stipend from the residency program's institution. The last two degrees are usually funded by a government agency.

Endodontics is an interesting field in that it deals exclusively with the dental pulp and surrounding tissues. The most common phrase that comes to mind is "root canal therapy." However, endodontics is a very lucrative field. Many general dentists don't have the time, skill, or other resources to deal with many of the endodontic type of problems that they will inevitably encounter, especially in teeth where the anatomy differs from the norm. The endodontist also performs certain types of surgery on tissues surrounding and involving the pulp. Endodontists may earn a Masters degree (MA or MS depending on the residency program), a doctorate, or a certificate. Endodontics residencies almost always require tuition to be paid by the dentist regardless of whether or not the dentist is on a degree or certificate track.

Oral and Maxillofacial Pathology is dentistry's version of the medical pathologist. Although most students don't especially love this area, it is nonetheless a very important one, especially in light of the dentist's expanding role from that of a technician to that of a diagnostician. Generally, oral pathologists are employed for research and as educators by learning institutions including dental and medical schools. Often, a general dentist, as well as a specialist, will send in a tissue sample that they suspect might be pathogenic to be analyzed by the oral pathologist. Oral pathologists may earn a Masters degree (usually MA), or a Doctor of Philosophy degree (PhD). Often, a residency program (sponsored by a few schools) will offer a stipend to the resident to offset the cost of tuition, which varies widely from program to program.

Oral and Maxillofacial Radiology is the newest specialty to be recognized by the ADA. In fact, approved in the fall of 1999, it is the newest dental specialty in 36 years (endodontics became recognized as a specialty in 1963). Currently, there are approximately 112 board-certified oral and maxillofacial radiologists. While the "job description" is somewhat in the formative stages, with all of the current practitioners working at hospitals and universities. This specialty will provide other dentists with an avenue of expert opinion, and will be available on a referral basis. In its press release, the ADA stated that oral and maxillofacial radiologists "will be able to assist general dentists and other oral health specialists in the diagnostic assessments of a range of diseases in the head and neck." While most dentists are proficient at interpreting radiographic images, they have little or no experience with advanced imaging technologies, such as CT scans and MRI images. As this information is being written, the details of the residency programs are being worked out. All eight of the programs that will offer a residency (six in the U.S., two in Canada), will require at least two years of post-doctoral education. It is likely that these programs will offer both a certificate and degree-granting tracks.

Perhaps the most lucrative, yet arguably most demanding field in dentistry, **Oral and Maxillofacial Surgery** involves the surgical intervention of oral and facial tissues due to oral diseases as well as for cosmetic reasons. Some common things that oral surgeons do include complicated tooth extractions, most notably, impacted third molars. Oral surgeons are also involved in removal of cancerous and precancerous lesions in the oral cavity along with other pathologies. Basic facial and jaw reconstruction are also within their domain. Oral surgeons must be competent with various types of sedation and complicated anesthetic techniques and principles. With further training, oral surgeons may obtain an M.D. degree, and even pursue plastic and other reconstructive surgical modalities. The downside of being an oral surgeon is that they tend to work a physician's hours. That is, they are burdened with being "on call" as well as working longer hours, often in a hospital setting. However, this lifestyle does appeal to many dental students, as does the increase in average yearly income. The degree tracks include Doctor of Medicine (MD), Masters degree (MA or MS depending on the program), a certificate, or a combination of any of the above. Oral surgery residency programs will pay a stipend usually over $30,000 for all four years. However, most programs that require or offer a MD degree will require a tuition payment for two years of medical school. Often, no stipend will be paid for the two years of medical school. Also, a combined MD/oral surgery certificate or Masters degree program will last at least 6 years, and more often, 7 years.

Orthodontics and Dentofacial Orthopedics is a field that deals mainly with changing the structural aspects of the oral environment. This includes the movement of teeth (orthodontics) and the movement of skeletal bone (orthopedics). Both techniques are essential to the achievement of a dentition and smile that is harmonious with other facial aspects. Because this field is so heavily geared towards cosmetics, although it does become involved with solving serious defects and other pathologies, cash flow is plentiful. Also, the work that an orthodontist does becomes less technically critical in the short term time frame. Rather, the work is more calculated to give the proper long term results. Because of the greater income and usually lighter physical style of work, this field tends to be the most competitive among the dental specialties. Like other clinical specialties, orthodontics residents are offered the option of a Masters degree (again, a MA or MS is dependent on the program), a doctorate, or a certificate. Like the endodontics residency, orthodontics residents pay a tuition to be trained. Some programs may offer some form of a stipend, but this is, by and large, not the case. A residency program may last from 2 to 3 years or more beyond dental school and depends on the program, as well as whether or not a Masters degree, PhD, or a certificate is the final objective.

Pediatric Dentistry is legally defined as dental work done on anyone less than 18 years of age. The specialty, however, goes much more in depth, involving psychological strategies of approaching the younger patient, and expertise with dental expectations and resolution of early dental and other oral diseases. Because the dental needs of children rarely involve some of the more complicated and time consuming procedures necessary in adult dental care, the amount of time spent per patient is less than it would otherwise be for an adult patient. Thus, the pediatric dentist may see as many as 80 patients in a single day whereas another specialist, such as a prosthodontist, may see less than 10 per day. Pediatric dentists also learn more complicated techniques involving sedation and anesthesia, as well as further training in dental treatment modalities chiefly involving dental concerns of children. This includes techniques from the fields of dental public health, orthodontics, and various operative techniques. Like orthodontics residents, pediatric dentistry residents have the option for a certificate or a Masters degree. Some programs even offer a doctoral degree. Although most programs provide a nice stipend, this can vary from program to program. Also, while some programs charge a tuition, but most programs will pay or waive for the student, any tuition requirements.

Periodontics is a changing field. In the past, it was referred to by many as "dentistry of the gums." While this is true, periodontists deal increasingly with those areas that were previously thought to be exclusive to the oral surgeon. Examples include bone augmentation of the mandible, surgical intervention in the oral cavity, and most recently, implantology. Although these changes will make a definite long term impact on the specialty, the bread and butter of periodontics is still surgical debridement of teeth and expertise with "gums." While this may not sound like an area that is in great demand, it is in fact a growing need. As the population ages and retains their teeth, there will be an ever increasing need for a periodontist's expertise in management of the soft tissues of the mouth. Most programs offer a certificate as well as a Masters degree. Some even offer a PhD degree, usually in an oral biological science. Residencies last from 2 to 3 years, and usually provide little or no financial compensation. Very few programs pay the resident a significant sum of money, but there are a few programs that do. The trend tends to be: the larger the financial compensation offered by a program, the more competitive it is to enter that particular program.

Prosthodontics is a field that may need a new job description. There are very few prosthodontists in the United States today, but no other profession has the expertise that affects so many Americans, especially as the population ages. With the advent of denturists, people who are able to manufacture and fit dentures in the absence of a dentist, it may seem that prosthodontists might be short on work. However, with the retirement of the baby boomers, it would be hard to see a situation where prosthodontists would not be in very high demand. Also, being experts in dental materials and esthetic reconstruction, skilled prosthodontists are among the few who are able to meet the demands of even the most difficult cases, in terms of both reconstruction of the dentition as well as high esthetic demands. Also, prosthodontists can sub-specialize as **maxillofacial prosthodontists**. These dentists design and manufacture the prostheses necessary to restore esthetics to patients who have undergone noticeable resection (surgical excision of pathological tissue, such as a cancer, a large cyst, or other aggressive form of disease) or other surgical intervention. For example, they may provide the nose, ear, eye, and a section of the palate and face for a patient that had to have those areas removed due to an accident, or more commonly, an invasive cancer. In addition to restoring the soft tissue aspects of a patient, the maxillofacial prosthodontist also restores their oral function. This may include being able to talk, as in the case of a person who has had their sinus invaded, or for patients who have cleft palate. Another function would be chewing. So, the maxillofacial prosthodontist adds teeth to a device that would be used to help the patient in other ways.

Recently, there has been a massive projected shortage of academic dentists. These dentists work for teaching or research institutions. In the next few years, you will see a concerted effort put forth by schools and governments to encourage and recruit dental students to consider a career in teaching and/or research. It is only logical that such a move would provide dental students with options to repaying their astronomical student loans, provide benefits packages that increase the worth of a teaching contract, along with other perks that would be needed to lure more dentists into teaching positions. Along these lines, an increasingly popular option to specializing is to obtain a Doctor of Philosophy degree in oral health sciences, or some other related field. This degree can coincide with, or be the culmination of a previous degree in a specialty. It can also be unrelated to any specific specialty, but instead be in a "generic" area of oral health sciences. Regardless of what path is taken to achieve this degree, such an endeavor would expose the dentist to scholarly research skills, and further equip them to better manage the transition to academic dentistry.

If this option seems appealing to you, then you should contact your prospective dental schools for more information. Some programs even offer joint DDS/PhD, or DMD/PhD degree programs. The advantage of this is a savings of time spent in obtaining the degrees, since working towards each degree independently of each other would require a longer period of study. Often, a school will require you to be admitted to both the pre-doctoral dental program (which would result in a DDS or DMD), and to the graduate program (which would result in a PhD). One thing to keep in mind when researching this area of dentistry, is that many of these joint degree programs are still in their formative stages. Thus, it may be up to you, prior to or during your interview, to ask about what type of "package" is offered by the school.

There are many other areas that are not recognized by the ADA as "official" specialties. Although they are not regulated or endorsed by the ADA, they are, nonetheless, available to the dental graduate. For example, recently there have been other "quasi" specialties that have emerged due to the increased need for dentists who are experts in areas that are not currently categorized in the list of specialties that exist today. There is a great likelihood that some of these areas will be incorporated in the near future as recognized specialties by the American Dental Association. A short list of these areas include dental anesthesiology, oral medicine, dental informatics, and dental jurisprudence. Other career opportunities that exist for dental graduates include dental insurance, dental materials research, dental technology research, manufacturing, and sales. Basically, the only limitations on what can be done is up to the imagination and specific interests of the dentist.

As you begin your dental experience, try to keep in mind the various opportunities that exist in the form of general dentistry, specialties, and "other" categories. This will enable you to measure your performance in a meaningful way, and also help you to have an idea of what is interesting to you. In your spare time, research the ins and outs of the various careers in dentistry. Know the job descriptions associated with each career, and ask questions to people in fields that you might be interested in.

2. How to Get There from Here

There are many paths that will eventually lead a person to dentistry. Some of those paths take longer than others, and there is, to be sure, a smarter path than most. That path, however, is not the same for everyone, and may involve different requirements depending on the situation of each individual. For example, the person who didn't realize that dentistry was, in fact, there life's goal, will take a longer path, but it might still be a smarter path than he or she may have otherwise taken. On the other hand, the person who opts not to graduate, but instead enters dental school after only two years of college, has taken the shortest path possible, but maybe not the smartest one. Perhaps this person will regret not having taken the opportunity to explore other careers. They may always feel unsure that dentistry was, in fact, the "right choice" for them. Therefore, the "best path" depends solely on who is doing what, and why they are doing it.

For most students pursuing a career in dentistry, the choice was not difficult. For various reasons, the profession seemed to suit them. There are many, however, who haven't even the vaguest of ideas as to why they chose dentistry. For these people, now is the time to find out what you're about to get yourself into. Four years of education beyond college is no small investment of time and money. Also, if it hasn't been publicized enough, dentistry along with other professional careers, may involve very high levels of stress that must be dealt with on a daily basis.

This may be due to a demanding workload, finances, managing other people, and other environmental and personal factors. For some, this translates into higher rates of suicide and unhappiness among the list of possible careers. While this is not unique to dentistry, it is still something that should be considered prior to choosing it as a career. The aspiring dental student should be prepared to pay his or her dues in order to reap the rewards of success.

There are a few requirements that must be met prior to being accepted into dental school. The requirements that do not change from school to school are: attending college for a minimum of two years, taking the four basic sciences prior to enrollment at dental school[2], and taking the DAT (Dental Admission Test) prior to enrollment at dental school. Requirements that may change depending on the school include: minimum grade point averages, minimum DAT scores, additional courses to be taken prior to enrollment (such as calculus, psychology, etc.), and preference given to in-state versus out-of-state residents (most publicly funded schools). The earlier this information sinks in, the better off you will be. If you wait too long to find out these requirements for the school in which you are interested, it may be too late. Phone numbers and addresses for each school are provided in *Appendix A*. Plan early in order to avoid the regret that so commonly accompanies those who wait until the last minute to find out this information.

---

[2]The four basic sciences are Biology, General Chemistry, Organic Chemistry, and General Physics. All four must include a lab section. While all four must be completed prior to enrollment, acceptance into a school does not require that all four have been completed, or even begun. Also, on the DAT exam, each of the basic sciences will be covered with the exception of Physics.

What to consider

Generally speaking, there are two major things that should be considered when applying to a dental school: first, are you going to specialize or practice as a general dentist? Second, how much does it cost? There are other factors that should also be weighed including, what type of environment will I be in (seasons, local climate, attitudes and beliefs such as social, political, religious, etc.)? Which school will be easiest to get into? Which school will keep me closest to my family and friends? There are many other personal factors that will and should influence the final decision of where to enroll, but none of these should take precedence over the two major factors mentioned above.

The question is often asked, "How do I know whether I'll want to specialize or not?" To know for certain is almost impossible, thus, attempting to get into the highest ranked school is often the end result. However, this may not be the wisest path to take. There are many who are pretty certain that they will become general dentists. This may be the result of a lifestyle choice-"I want to take it easy in dental school and just graduate and get my license." A practical decision-"I know my limits, and I know that almost 80% of dentists will be general dentists. I also want to start earning money as soon as possible, and the location that I want to practice in doesn't need a specialist." On the other hand, there are those who are quite certain that they would like to pursue a specialty. This conclusion is usually based on personal experience and research into a particular specialty area. Thus, those with an informed decision will say, "I've looked into it, and I am certain that specializing is in my best interests, and I'm willing to sacrifice my resources to study harder and longer than most other students." Others will decide to forego specialization using similar arguments to those mentioned previously. Unfortunately, most people will fall somewhere in the grayer areas-"I'm not sure if I want to or not, so I'll apply to the highest ranked schools I can and see what happens." All of these are valid conclusions, but the ones who know one way or the other if they will specialize or not, are going to be the ones who will find a school that suits them the best. It is important to keep in mind that there is no official ranking system of dental schools. Rather, a magazine, or other form of private entity, will rank schools according to various criteria. Of course, it can generally be said that these rankings, though not official in nature, paint a pretty good picture of where a particular institution stands relative to their peers.

By knowing if you will specialize or not, the list of potential schools that you will look at can be shortened. If you choose to specialize, then a school that emphasizes or is renowned for the specialty that you are interested in would be an obvious contender. Also, most of the top ten institutions would serve your ultimate purposes well. This is because a higher ranked school will be to your benefit when it comes time to match with a residency program. While there are graduates from every dental school who will pursue a specialty, the percentage of those at higher ranked institutions who will apply for a specialty position and who get accepted into a program will be greater. A proper analogy would be: similar students in terms of test scores, grade point averages, and class ranking apply to a dental school. Student A graduates from Tinyville College. Student B graduates from Big Ivy University. Who is going to be accepted over the other? Similarly, when applying to a residency program the determining factor between similarly ranked students with similar qualifying credentials will most likely be the school from which each student graduates. So, for those who want to specialize, it is very important to attend a higher ranked school. Conversely, for those who know they want to practice as a general dentist, ranking becomes secondary to other factors that may be more important at the moment. Remember that these are generalizations. There will always be those students that will not fall under this example. However, in most situations, the example mentioned above will be applicable.

For the student who is rather sure that they will not be specializing, schools that emphasize complete and thorough clinical training should top their list. While all accredited schools meet *minimum* requirements, some just have better access than others, especially in terms of the patient pool. For example, a highly ranked institution located in a more rural setting is less likely to cater to overall technical and clinical needs than a lower ranked school that is nestled in the heart of a big city. This is just a fact. Therefore, if general practice is the ultimate goal, seek advice from local dentists who have graduated from various schools. Ask them if their program was catered more towards academics and research, or towards emphasizing mastery of the technical, operative, and restorative aspects of dentistry. This decision for a more "practical" school will result in greater operator skill and speed in the first few years out of dental school compared to graduates of schools that are more academic or research oriented.

Be warned! Regardless of what school you go to, higher ranked or lower ranked, when it comes time to getting into a residency for a specialty, the most important factor is usually your class ranking within your own dental school class. Other factors are also important, such as national board scores, research involvement and publications, professional experiences, among other things. Therefore, be ready to compete near the top of the class no matter where you go. Although there is some leeway given to students from programs that are recognizably more difficult due to the institution and the caliber of students attending there, relative class standing is still very important. In fact, this may be a reason for someone seeking to specialize to attend a lower ranked institution, where there may be a better chance of graduating with a higher class ranking. This is an assumption based on the lower entering class averages at lower ranked schools, thus, there may be a lower level of competition from other members of the class. This is, however, very much a gamble. There is no way to know for certain that a class will be less competitive. Therefore, it is probably a better idea to attend a more highly ranked school than to take any unnecessary risks.

Cost

The cost of education is astounding. The cost of dental education is even more amazing. The average amount of debt incurred by a graduating dental student averages around $80,000, and is increasing every year. Some students even have loan amounts exceeding $200,000 from dental school alone! Few realize this, and even fewer plan ahead, thinking that when the money flows in after graduation, everything will be just fine. This might be the case if the dental school loan is the only one that exists. However, most students have some or all of their undergraduate loans still outstanding, and what about the loan to establish a private practice? The two biggest areas of loans associated with dentistry are school related loans and business related loans. Both must be approached with caution in order to minimize their long term effects. Thus, a simple solution would be to attend a state university instead of a private institution. This may not always be the case, however, as residency requirements and other unforseen costs may become associated with some situations. Nevertheless, in most cases, a state supported dental school will be at least $10,000 cheaper to attend. So, practically speaking, the less money spent on education, the less needed to repay when it comes time to start making payments.

In terms of cost, if someone is entering dental school with great certainty that he or she will not specialize, then it is only logical that finding the most affordable education is in his or her best interests. It makes no sense to pay more, only to find that the education and experience was not so different from the one offered at a school with a more affordable level of tuition. This is especially true in regard to the amount of dental educational loans that will burden the dental graduate, as mentioned above. When deciding which dental schools should appear on a short list, it behooves the undergraduate who is seeking admission into dental school, to find out more about the details of the school or schools that appear on his or her list of potential choices. A price-performance evaluation needs to be done in order to choose the school that will satisfy your interests. Too many students just take whatever is handed to them, only to later regret their lack of active involvement in the careful evaluation of their needs as well as the facts and figures associated with any potential schools. What may have been a necessity at the time of enrollment, later transforms into a mountain of debt and worry, especially when it comes time to start making those first payments on a huge student loan that continues to snowball due to constantly accruing interest.

Finally, most applicants will not have much more than a vague idea of whether or not specializing lies within their career goals. The only solution to this is to study the options and observe specialists in your immediate area. Most dentists are more than happy to speak to a pre-dental club, or to allow observation by a student who is interested in learning more about dentistry. This applies to general dentists and specialists alike. The best thing to do is to have a pre-dental club representative contact the dentist or specialist and arrange for a presentation or lecture. Arranging personal observation times should be no problem at this point. If school is out, or you don't have access to a pre-dental club, then just call the doctor, explain your interests, and he or she will usually be willing to set up a time for you to come in. Often, especially when the dentist is busy, you may not get through. In that case, having a professor write or call the office will help. Whatever you do, don't give up. Remember, it will only help you to know more about the field which you are about to become a part of.

3. The Measurements: Your GPA and the DAT

Every school has a minimum GPA and DAT score that is required for admission. In the last few years, although the minimums have not changed much, the average statistics of the applicants and enrollees have progressively increased. That is, what used to be an average GPA of 3.2 at a particular school may now be 3.4. The same goes for the DAT scores. When applying to a particular school, be sure that you at least know the minimum requirements for admission as well as any recent trends in that school's enrollee statistics. Otherwise, you will be wasting your money, since the admissions committee will not look beyond the front page of your application. The best way to get this information is to contact the prospective school. If this is not possible or desirable, then the information can be found in the book, *The ADEA Official Guide to Dental Schools* (former title: *Admission Requirements of U.S. and Canadian Dental Schools*), published by the American Dental Education Association. In it, you will find the minimum requirements of every dental school, along with other important information regarding each school.

Your GPA

The grade point average is often the casualty of a fun-filled, or "formative," undergraduate education. Many students who choose dentistry as their profession have majored in a science degree, which by its nature, tends to be tougher and more time consuming than other fields of study. Because of this, their GPA may have suffered. These students will generally have a difficult time being admitted into a top ten university. For those applicants with high averages, admittance to the dental school of their choice is much easier. Generally speaking, a grade point average of 3.50 and higher on a 4 point scale, is guaranteed admission to at least one of the top ten dental schools. This guarantee, however, hinges on the student's performance on the DAT, and the impression left at the interview. For most people who receive marks of this caliber, the DAT is merely a confirmation of their performance in college, and the interview a formality. Keep in mind, however, that a poor showing on the DAT, or a foolish remark or sloppy appearance at an interview may easily compromise what should have been a very comfortable position.

Since GPA is such a big factor in admissions, it would be wise to choose majors, or classes, that are familiar to you or subjects that are otherwise "easy." This is especially true immediately prior to submitting an application form. If you have any friends who have been accepted to medical school, you will notice that they really enjoy life in their last semester or two of school. This is because once a student is admitted, the only thing that can keep them out of that school in terms of academics, is a failing grade or some form of unethical behavior. If your GPA is struggling, save your "hard" classes for later (assuming that this is even an option for you), so that your GPA will be at its highest when you apply, not after you graduate. If your GPA is not so admirable, consider taking lots of easier classes to boost it prior to the application process.

Doubtless, there are some you by now, who are beginning to feel as if your earlier blunders or inexperience may have already cost you your chances to prove that you are a worthy candidate for admission into dental school.

There is some encouraging news! The DAT can be a lifesaver when it comes to "validating" a student. For example, perhaps general chemistry was not exactly your best subject, or you decided to leave early on vacation, missing your final exam. Whatever the circumstances, let's say that you end up with a C, or a 2.00 on a 4 point scale for the semester. When you took the DAT, however, by some stroke of luck or through hard work, you scored in the 95th percentile! It would be very difficult for an admissions committee not to take note of that high score. It "validates" the student by contradicting a poor mark. Usually, a good DAT score will help to reaffirm a student's potential and ability in the face of an otherwise lackluster grade point average. There are other tips and tricks to consider when taking the DAT, especially when getting a high score is imperative to your plight.

The DAT

So, how do you score higher on the DAT? Better yet, what is the DAT? DAT stands for "Dental Admission Test." It is operated by the American Dental Association, and is now available only on computer at authorized testing centers. The DAT is comprised of two sections: the Academic section, and the Perceptual Abilities section. The Academic section can be broken down to three sections: Survey of Natural

Sciences, Quantitative Reasoning, and Reading Comprehension. The Basic Sciences section can be further broken down into three subsections, although they will not be taken separately. They are: Biology, Inorganic Chemistry, and Organic Chemistry. See *Figure 1* for a breakdown of the sections. Let's take a look at each section and their respective subsections beginning with the Basic Sciences section.

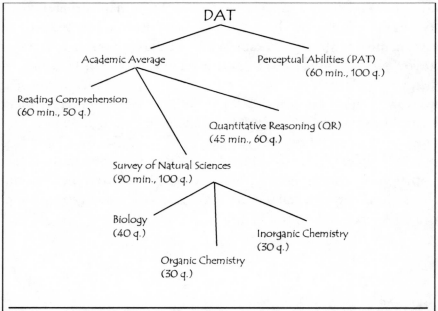

Figure 1. Note that min. refers to the number of minutes given for a section, and q. stands for he number of questions in a section.

Basic Sciences involves three of the four disciplines that are required for admission to any dental school: biology, general chemistry, and organic chemistry. Note that physics is not on the exam, thus it would be wise to leave physics as a subject that will be taken last among the four basic sciences, or if it is a difficult subject for you, taken in the last year of school prior to entering dental school. A list of the basic areas that will be covered in the biology portion of the basic sciences section of the exam can be found in *Table 1*. Inorganic chemistry topics are listed in *Table 2*. Organic chemistry topics are listed in *Table 3*.

Scoring well on the DAT is a confirmation of a strong GPA. High scores also "validate" a mediocre undergraduate performance. Therefore, it is imperative that you score as high as possible on this examination. There are many ways to study for this exam. The first method is to purchase a review book and sample tests to familiarize yourself with the test and the format used to administer it. The second method is to enroll in a test preparation program, such as those offered by Kaplan, or the Princeton Review. The third method is to review old course materials. Of these three, the last is the least desirable path to take. This is due to the fact that you will probably not be reviewing aspects of the DAT that are critical to achieving higher scores. Furthermore, you will have no experience with the perceptual ability portion of the DAT. Finally, you will have "overstudied" for the survey of natural sciences section of the exam, as there can only be 100 questions, which will be from focused, topical areas. While the second method is a sure way to receive some form of comprehensive review and introduction to the DAT, it is also very expensive. Costs can be as high as $1000 to participate in this structured, guided form of review. Often times, these courses will be self taught, with books and videos as the student's only instructors. In fact, qualified DAT instructors who have taken and performed well on the test are in short supply. In some parts of the country, there are only a couple of instructors in a given state, if there are any at all.

The first method ("do-it-yourself") will be detailed in the next chapter. This method is very affordable ($100-$200), but it is up to you to have the motivation to start and complete the review process. If you know that you do not have the motivation to study on your own, then it is encouraged that you take the test preparation path to prepare yourself for the DAT. Otherwise, it is the most cost effective and, in our opinion, helpful, to follow the "do-it-yourself" method.

Table 1. Major topics of the biological sciences portion of the survey of natural sciences section of the DAT.

origin of life
cell metabolism and photosynthesis
enzymology
thermodynamics
organelle structures and function
biological organization and relationship of major
    taxa using the five-kingdom system
structure and function of vertebrate systems
  integumentary
  skeletal
  muscular
  circulatory
  immunological
  digestive
  respiratory
  urinary
  nervous
  endocrine
  reproductive

fertilization
descriptive embryology
developmental mechanics
Mendelian inheritance
chromosomal genetics
meiosis
molecular and human genetics
natural selection
population genetics
speciation
population and community ecology
animal behavior
  social behavior

Table 2. Major topics of the inorganic chemistry portion of the survey of natural sciences section of the DAT.

stoichiometry
   percent of composition
   empirical formulas from % of composition
   balancing equations
   weight/weight problems
   weight/volume problems
   density problems
gases
   kinetic molecular theory of gases
   Graham's, Dalton's, Boyle's, Charles laws
   ideal gas law
liquids and solids
solutions
   colligative properties
   concentration calculations
acids and bases
chemical equilibrium
   molecular
   acid/base
   precipitation and equilibrium calculations
thermodynamics and thermochemistry
   laws of thermodynamics
   Hess' law
   spontaneity prediction

chemical kinetics
   rate laws
   activation energy
   half life
oxidation-reduction reactions
   balancing equations
   determination of oxidation numbers
   electro-chemical concepts and calculations
atomic and molecular structure
   electron configuration
   orbital types
   Lewis-Dot diagrams
   atomic theories
   molecular geometry
   bond types
   quantum mechanics
periodic properties
   categories of non-metals
   transition metals
   non-transition metals
nuclear reactions

Table 3. Major topics of the organic chemistry portion of the survey of natural sciences section of the DAT.

bonding
  atomic orbitals
  molecular orbitals
  hybridization
  Lewis structures
  bond angles
  bond lengths
mechanisms
  energetics
  structure and stability of intermediates
  SN1 and SN2
  E1 and E2
  addition
  free radical and substitution mechanisms
chemical and physical properties of molecules
  stability
  solubility
  polarity
  inter- and intra-molecular forces
  separation techniques
organic analysis
  intro. infrared and 1H NMR spectroscopy
  simple chemical tests
stereochemistry
  conformational analysis
  optical activity
  chirality
  chiral centers
  places of symmetry
  enantiomers
  diasteriomers
  meso compounds

nomenclature
  IUPAC rules
  identification of functional groups
reaction of the major functional groups
  prediction of reaction products
  important mechanistic generalities
acid-base chemistry
  resonance effects
  inductive effects
  prediction of products
  equilibria
aromatic
  concept of aromaticity
  electrophilic aromatic substitution
  synthesis
  identification of the product of a simple
sequence reaction
  identification of the reagents

4. Tips and Tricks for the DAT

The DAT is like every other standardized test in that your main goal is to score high. As with other tests, there are two things that stand in your way. First, and foremost, is time. Because this test is timed, there will some parts or sections that you may not be able to complete. Second, is knowledge of the material. The survey of natural sciences section is based on knowledge that you should have learned in your prerequisite undergraduate science courses. Quantitative reasoning and reading comprehension are subjects that every college student should be familiar with, and are tested at a school difficulty level. Both of these sections are similar to the math and verbal sections on other college entrance examinations. The perceptual ability section is the only part of the exam that is truly unique to the DAT. In this section you will find diagrams and figures that must be mentally manipulated in order to find a correct answer.

So, how should you study for this exam? The method that will be discussed here will be the "do-it-yourself" method. The other two methods, mentioned in the previous chapter, are also available. For a structured, lecture-based review, look in your phone book's yellow pages under "test preparation," or refer to the "Additional Resources" chapter of this book. The other method is to review all of your class notes, and to read the course book in its entirety. This last method is strongly discouraged because it involves too much time and effort on your part to score as high as these other two methods will allow. For all three of these options, as a pre-dental student, you will find that there is a massive shortage of any material relating to pre-doctoral admissions to dental school. When it comes to the DAT, there is even less information. This applies even to the expensive test preparation courses. Keep in mind, that just knowing what the test is about, knowing the rules, and knowing the time limits, will all help you to automatically score higher on the DAT. Before spending close to $1000, ask someone who has taken a test preparation course about their own experiences. Then ask someone who has taken the DAT with only self-study, using materials that are available in most bookstores, about their opinions. Either way, you can keep up to date, via the web site *www.predentalinfo.com*, of any new and worthwhile publications to help you in your preparations for the DAT.

A complete review of the survey of natural sciences is beyond the scope of this book, especially since there are several excellent review books already on the market. These books are written for review of the MCAT, the entrance examination for medical school. However, these texts adequately cover the vast majority of material that will appear on the DAT. These texts are listed both in the "Additional Resources" chapter of this book, as well as on the Pre-Dental Info web site, *www.predentalinfo.com*.

There is a true lack of materials for preparation of the perceptual abilities portion of the DAT. Currently, there are only two adequate review materials available. First, the application packet for the DAT, which contains an excellent example of the real DAT. Second, is the Top Score DAT simulation software. The latter is listed in this book, and both are available through the Pre-Dental Info web site, for your convenience.

The first thing you should do is to order a review book listed in the "Additional Resources" chapter of this book. If you'd rather take a hands on look at the choices, go to your local bookstore and find the recommended titles. Take time to browse through the book, finding the style of presentation that you think would best suit you. Basically, a good MCAT review book is what you should be looking for. This will cover the vast majority of basic science material that you need to know for the DAT. When looking for a book that is not on our list of recommended titles, pay close attention to the major subject areas covered within it. Do this by comparing the table of contents of a prospective book with *Tables 1, 2,* and *3,* which can be found at the end of Chapter 3 of this book. Remember to frequently visit the Prothotech web site, for up to the minute information on the best available books and other test preparation resources. Other titles that are recommended will help you understand the perceptual abilities portion of the examination, as well as the reading comprehension and quantitative analysis sections. Keep in mind that the PAT section is the most poorly covered area of the DAT exam in terms of truly helpful review materials. Be careful when choosing a PAT review book, and be sure to first evaluate the recommendations that are made in Chapter 6.

Let's take a look at each section of the exam. First, the survey of natural sciences. This section has three portions: biology, inorganic chemistry, and organic chemistry. To begin with, you must have a review book to guide you to the important points concerning the various topics. Most review books have their own tailored way of helping you to accomplish this task. Most of their suggestions are worthwhile, but keep in mind that there are both good and bad ways to study for each of these components. *Always remember* that the test can ask you only 40 questions for biology, 30 questions for inorganic chemistry, and 30 questions for organic chemistry. Just take a look at your basic sciences textbooks. Each one has at least 20-30 major topic areas. It is only logical that the DAT will *never* ask more than two or three questions per topic. There is no space or time on the exam to ask any more than this! This means that when you study, try to spread things out. Don't try to memorize every detail of every process, unless it is specifically mentioned on the tables in Chapter 3 of this book, or unless you see a similar question on a practice test. This will help you to focus your attention and resources on the types of questions that will most likely be asked on the exam. Remember, just 40 questions for biology, 30 questions for inorganic chemistry, and 30 questions for organic chemistry. Always refer back to the tables in Chapter 3 to force yourself to stay on track with the topics that you will most likely be tested on.

Another piece of advice to contemplate, is to focus on areas in which you are weak. Too often, students will review material that they are virtually experts on. They always answer correctly on questions pertaining to this material, yet they continue to study and review it. This is a total waste of precious time. Many of you will procrastinate until the last minute to review for the DAT. For you, this little piece of advice is a gem. Not only do you have very little time to review for the test, you may not even be familiar with the basics let alone the details of the exam. Start by taking a practice test. This applies to everyone. Don't time yourself! The important thing is to keep track of the question *types* that are foreign to you. This means, the topics that you've forgotten, the formulas you don't know, math problems in which you are weak, and perceptual ability rules that you don't understand. This will provide you with a map of things that require priority attention. Over the next few days, concentrate on understanding and memorizing the information, concepts, formulas, and rules for each of these types of problem areas. You will have a much better chance of answering a question that you know something about, as opposed to if you had not known anything at all. For the questions that you had little or no difficulty answering–you don't have the time to keep rehashing information that you already know! The odds are very much in your favor, that you will answer these types of questions correctly if and when they are presented to you. Of course, this is assuming that you really do understand the concepts and information behind the question to begin with.

Review of the Natural Sciences

The "best" way to study for the **biology** portion is to review and memorize the major topics found under each of the areas listed in *Table 1*. This simple instruction cannot be overemphasized! There will be a few concepts that will appear as biology questions. These are major concepts based on the topics listed in that table. The vast majority, if not all, of the questions will be based on these major topics and subject headings.

From past experience, the "favorites" include questions on: enzymes, differences in the structures of prokaryotic and eukaryotic cells, eukaryotic organelles and their various functions, cell division or mitosis, a few questions on taxonomy under the five kingdoms, several questions on vertebrate systems, sexual reproduction including fertilization and meiosis, Mendelian inheritance and chromosomal genetics (phenotypes and alleles, dominant vs. recessive), evolutionary concepts (natural selection, population principles), and learned behavior vs. instincts. There will always be questions related to these principles on every DAT examination. Focus your review on these topics as they are guaranteed to show up on the examination. Finally, make sure that you know the specific topics listed in *Table 1*, as any topical questions on the exam that are not specifically mentioned here will come from that list.

For enzymes, know the principles of activation and positive vs. negative feedback as well as the terms associated with enzymes in general such as: allosteric or conformational, coenzymes, catalysis, activation energy, substrate, and conservation of enzymes.

When you study the cell, know the similarities and differences between a prokaryote and a eukaryote. Which one has a nucleus? How do they replicate? What kind of genetic material is found in each? How are their enzymes and other proteins manufactured? What types of organelles are found in each cell? What kind of cells are plants, and what makes them unique? What is an anaerobe? An aerobe? What's the difference between a facultative anaerobe and a strict anaerobe? These are the areas that the DAT will cover, so knowing the answers to these questions will prepare you for this topic.

Cell division or mitosis questions are geared towards eukaryotic cells. You should still know the various ways in which prokaryotic cells and fungi reproduce. Know the four phases of the cell cycle. Know about the phases of mitosis and what happens in each one. Know the differences between mitosis and meiosis. Other topics may include cancer cell replication, and microtubular structure and arrangement.

The system of taxonomy in biology is something you will just have to memorize. Know the major kingdoms and their subsequent categories. There will be a few questions that will require that you know the levels of classification and which titles go with a specific category. The good thing is that the questions have traditionally been on an animal that is pretty distinctive, such as a starfish or lobster.

The major functional systems common to vertebrates should be looked at in depth. Your review book will have detailed schematics and explanations of these systems. Pay close attention to the muscular, respiratory, circulatory, digestive, and immunological systems. The other systems listed in *Table 1* are also fair game. While understanding concepts is important in this section, the questions will be rather specific, so memorizing terms and characteristics is equally important to this section.

Sexual reproduction questions will mainly involve the area of human reproduction, although, as mentioned above, knowing how other organisms reproduce is crucial (bacteria, fungi, and plants). Know the sequence and phases of meiosis and how it is different in mitosis. Know the process and importance of genetic crossover that occurs in meiosis. Know the differences between male and female gametogenesis (oogenesis vs. spermatogenesis) and the number of gametes that result from this process. Know the cycle and window of opportunity for fertilization in the female, and the time line associated with pregnancy. Know what makes a male a male, and a female a female.

Classical genetics and Mendel's laws will be covered in the exam, as well as several questions on chromosomal genetics. Know how to do a Punnett square and the outcomes for the various paternal and maternal combinations. Know the concept of phenotypes and how it relates to the concept of dominant vs. recessive genes. Understand the various types of inheritance: autosomal recessive, autosomal dominant, and x-linked or sex-linked recessive. Know the concepts of blood typing, and how to predict blood types given parental antibody/antigen combinatoins. Finally, know the five conditions of the Hardy-Weinberg principle of genetic frequency, as it is almost always on the DAT exam.

You should be familiar with the basics of animal behavior, such as the various types of conditioning. Also, know the concepts of natural selection, population genetics (and formulas), ecology, and plant biology. This last category is very important, in that it interrelates with so many other topics. Understanding these various relationships will further prepare you for the exam.

Inorganic chemistry is a subject that eludes many people. It is not something that you can just pick up, study, and understand well enough to be prepared for the DAT. Therefore, when reviewing for this portion of the test, try to approach the material in a "building block" manner. That is, before moving on to a new topic, make sure you fully understand the principles that are covered in the topic that you're leaving, assuming that it is related with subsequent material. Most people make the common mistake of trying to memorize pages of formulas and numbers for this section. This is a complete waste of time. Generally speaking, if you don't understand the governing principle behind a problem, no formula or number will ever help you. Instead of filling your brain with lots of stuff to remember, try to study for this by recognizing what is going on. There are a few things that should be memorized, but this is in the sense of being familiar with the terminology and definitions involved in the broader principles.

For example, there is always a question on nuclear chemistry. There are a lot of things that you *could* memorize. However, the questions will almost always involve some basic principles about the subject. Beyond a firm grasp of the idea of half-lives, they will ask for you to fill in simple variables involving a nuclear reaction such as:

$$^{12}_{6}C \longrightarrow ^{0}_{+1}e^{+} \underline{\hspace{2cm}}$$

When you understand that the carbon 12 (six neutrons) is emitting a positron (one proton), you know that the resulting atom would be nitrogen 12 (seven neutrons). So, the important thing to know in this question was the general process of nuclear decay and radiation. The only thing you had to memorize were the definitions of alpha, beta, gamma rays, and a positron.

Past questions on the inorganic chemistry portion of the exam, have covered the material listed in *Table 2*. Stoichiometric questions are always on the exam. Know how to balance equations, and how to determine molecular formulas from percent compositions, and vice versa. Density is another topic that is often covered.

Review of gases should focus on the ideal gas law. Remember, complex calculations, or other form of gross time consumption is not the intention of this portion of the DAT. Rather, it is to see what amount of objective information that you are aware of. So, knowing the ideal gas law, and how it relates to practically every other gas law, is essential. You may not be asked a computational type of question, but you may see questions that will ask for the principles behind certain conditions.

For liquids and solids, know the various phase change diagrams, and especially the triple point diagram. Also, be familiar with the various terms associated with each diagram. Know the colligative changes, and what types of compounds will cause the greatest effects. Know how to calculate concentration, and also what the differences are, and how to convert between molarity and molality.

Know the various types of acids and bases, and how they are defined. Be able to identify weak and strong acids and bases. Know how to calculate pH and pOH values for a given acid or base. Know other types of chemical equations: hot to write them, how to balance them, how to calculate equilibrium, yield, and saturation.

For thermodynamics, familiarize yourself with the laws of thermodynamics, entropy, enthalpy, various definitions and terms related to heat, and several basic approaches to calculating changes in heat such as Hess' law. Know the differences between heat of formation and heat of reaction, as well as, the methods of calculating net heat gain or loss from a chemical equation. Related to liquids and solids, know how to calculate total changes in heat when going from a liquid to a solid, or from a solid to a liquid, the differences between exothermic and endothermic reactions, and know how to convert from calories to Joules. Finally, know when a given reaction will be spontaneous, and when it won't.

For chemical kinetics, understand rate laws, and how to determine the various orders of a reaction, given pertinent experimental data. Also, know how catalysts work, what they do to the activation energy, what they do to the net change in energy, and whether or not they are used up in a reaction. Chemical half-lives are also a topic that may come up. Know the application of this term as it relates to chemical reactions, as opposed to nuclear half-lives.

Oxidation-reduction reactions can cause many people to stumble. Therefore, be very familiar with the identification and naming of the reactants and products, and be able to balance a given red-ox reaction.

The basics of inorganic chemistry will also be covered. These include: the atom and its structure, writing and recognizing electron configurations, knowing the various orbital types, being able to draw and recognize a Lewis-Dot diagram, knowing the basic atomic theories and principles, knowing the common angles and other bond geometry found in all molecules, and a solid understanding of quantum mechanics. Knowing his last topic will help you to understand some of the basic principles of the periodic table, such as how the various elements are grouped. Beyond that, you must know how to identify metals and non-metals, and know their respective characteristics. Be aware of trends in the periodic table when going up, down, left and right. These trends should include: electronegativity, mass, atomic radius, ionization energy, and number of free orbitals. Know how to identify a covalent versus an ionic compound. Know the idiosyncracies of the transition metals, and how they relate to the non-transition metals. Also, know the basic intermolecular forces and be able to recognize them. Finally, know how to identify an element and the meanings of the various numbers associated with an element.

Organic chemistry should be studied like a combination of biology and inorganic chemistry. The key principles, like steric hindrance, chirality, intermolecular bond types, and electronegativity will help you to understand what is going on in the hundreds of reactions that you are expected to be familiar with. For example, by understanding steric hindrance, you can differentiate between SN and E type reactions. When it comes to picking a specific type of reaction, for a specific reactant in a particular solution, knowing this will be important. It's not that you will be asked a direct question on the principle, but knowing the how and why, will save you from having to memorize many of the less important reactions.

The subject of bonding encompasses many important concepts. These include orbitals, hybridization, bond angles, and bond lengths.

Know how to estimate the bond angles and bond lengths from a given molecular structure. Know what affects these properties. Memorize the basic geometrical structures and the various types of bonds that are associated with them.

Know the principles of stability, solubility, and polarity. Know the various factors that influence each of these, such as the intramolecular and intermolecular forces, functional groups, size of the molecule, etc. Know the major intermolecular forces, and be able to rank various types of molecules "in order" when they differ in functional groups, length, etc. Know the basics of separation techniques, such as distillation, filtration, and electrical separation. Be aware of the principles of infrared and NMR spectroscopy. The more important one for this test will be the infrared spectroscopy. Therefore, be familiar with the areas where specific groups will be found. Also, know how these areas can be affected by other factors.

Stereochemistry is a major subject that you should understand very well. Questions regarding this material will be based on concepts, and will usually involve locating chiral centers, identifying meso compounds, enantiomers, diasteriomers, and other isomeric combinations. Know how to determine whether a compound is R or S. Know when a compound is optically active, and it what scenarios a compound or a solution will be optically inactive. Understand how to differentiate between the various types of isomers when viewing a 3-dimensional diagram or a Fischer projection.

The IUPAC naming scheme is critically important to know and understand. Several questions will arise that will require you to know this system in and out. Keep in mind that there is much information that goes into naming a molecule including: axial versus equatorial positions, R and S naming rules, rules involving double and triple bonds, being able to identify and properly name the many functional groups, and prioritizing all of the above. Know how the functional groups affect a reaction, and how they are important in the prediction of the products of a reaction. Know how they relate to intermolecular forces, and how they affect the intramolecular stability and tendencies of a molecule.

Know how to identify an aromatic compound, as this is a topic that is a DAT favorite. Know which compounds are traditional "traps" and which ones appear like "traps," but are, in fact, actual aromatics. Understand the reactions leading to aromatic synthesis, and be able to identify the products and reagents used in simple aromatic reactions.

There are many reactions that should be memorized. To list all of them would be redundant, as they are easily accessed through one of the recommended review books.

To recap, try to remain focused on the tables listed in chapter 3. They will keep you from studying material that may not even be on the test. When purchasing a basic science review book, keep in mind the "favorite" areas mentioned above that the DAT likes to cover.

Time Management

The most important asset that any test taker has, is confidence. Confidence can be gained through practice, and familiarity with the test material. As with any talent or skill that is recognized only when exhibited under pressure, confidence needs to rest on a firm foundation of practice, more practice, and even more practice. However, there are some simple concepts that are often overlooked by many test takers. These are basic principles that can be applied to any test, and don't require as great of a commitment and dedication to practice as does attaining a rock hard level of confidence. The two most important principles are: time management and good guessing. By now, I'm sure you've had your share of sagacious advice on *how* to take a standardized test. You probably even have your own techniques to succeed. If these techniques that you've learned or come up with are consistently resulting in high standardized test scores, then by all means, please continue to use them. If, however, you are like most people, a little advice wouldn't hurt.

Time management involves many factors. Proper time management requires you to sit down and become a general, planning the attack before committing any resources, and properly designating those resources as soon as a solid plan has been conceived. This means that you must know your enemy. Regarding time management, your enemy is anything that slows you down or keeps you from completing the examination in a comfortable fashion. Let's start from the top.

The first thing that you should do is to set a goal for yourself. This is a very subjective task. While one score may be acceptable for you, it may be unacceptable for others. It is our recommendation that you set a realistic goal, or score, that you think will be respectable in the eyes of the schools to which you plan on applying to. In terms of the DAT, this score will be anywhere from 1 to 30, with 1 being the lowest score possible, and 30 being the highest. Next, raise your target score by two or three points. So, if you think a 17 on the academic portion of the exam will be a good score, you should add 2 arriving at 19, or 3 to arrive at 20. Thus, 19 or 20 will be your new target score. The reason for this is that when preparing for this test, a higher score will cause you aim higher. In all of your practice work, you should not be satisfied with anything less than the elevated goal. This sets a bar, that if reached, will add immensely to your credentials. If you happen to fall short of that goal, you will still be in the range, and probably above the initial goal that you had set. Too many dental school candidates just want to achieve the minimum or average scores to get in. This is a poor attitude to foster, especially in an increasingly competitive admissions process.

Next, take a practice exam. The best preliminary test to use is the sample DAT that is provided with your DAT application packet. For now, forget about time. Time management is a skill that will be gained and exercised with other resources. For now, the most important thing, is to know your weak points and your strong points. After identifying the general subject areas in which you are weak, take a closer look and pinpoint specific areas in which you are deficient. This is hard to do from looking at one practice test. Therefore, view this as an ongoing process. As you use more resources to help you gain experience for the DAT, always try to identify areas in which you are consistently strong, and more importantly, consistently weak.

After this, focus your attention on *why* you are weak in a particular area. Are you a slow reader? Are you unprepared for the biology portion of the exam? Are you unfamiliar with the instructions for the PAT? Are you rusty with your math skills? Whatever the cause, be sure to note it, and to do something about it. Try a different method of reading. Focus on reviewing material dealing with biology. Carefully read and understand what is expected of you on the PAT. Ask others for help with equations that you're having problems with. At the same time, spend a little less time reviewing for the areas in which you know that you are strong. If you know it, you know it! However, if you still feel a little shaky with a subject, you should try to hone that area until you are consistent. This should not be done, however, until you have finished strengthening your weaker areas. You will know that you have reached your potential when you are achieving a consistent score. At this point, the wisest course of action would be to make your strong areas even stronger. By doing this, you will be arming yourself with the information and techniques that allow you to answer basic questions and question types in categories that you would otherwise be lost. This will increase your chances of answering a greater number of questions correctly, instead of trying to squeeze a few more correct responses from areas in which you are already scoring well. As you will see, a few points in your weakest areas will make a tremendous difference in the final analysis.

Another thing to keep in mind, is that the survey of natural sciences is not too bad when it comes to time management. Rather, scoring well on this section requires knowledge of the material. However, with the DAT now an exclusively computerized exam, adequate time management may become a problem for some of you. To combat this for all sections of the DAT, there are a few things that you can do to maximize the time you have to actually spend on the exam. When you arrive to take your test, you will be given some scratch paper. On that paper, make a few grids similar to an account ledger. In *Figure 2*, you will see one example of a simple grid. In this grid, you will see the answer choices A through E written across the top, and the question number that is undecided is written along the left side. As you encounter a question for which you just can't seem to decide on an answer, write the number along the left hand side, and place an "x" in the boxes that correspond to the answer choices that you have determined are incorrect. Also, be sure to guess on an answer before moving on. If time runs out, you will at least have an answer marked down instead of having nothing. Also, this answer will have been based on your hunch at the time you initially encountered the question, which by the way, is the best time for a hunch-based response.

	A	B	C	D	E
3	X	X			
17		X	X	X	
22					X
23		X		X	
34			X		X

In this example, the test-taker has had some difficulty with question #3. So far, she has eliminated answer choices A and B, and crossed out the spaces corresponding to the question and eliminated answer choices. Jumping to question #22, she has only eliminated one answer choice, in this case E, and has crossed out the corresponding space. From this example, the value of utilizing a grid should be obvious. This grid will help you to keep track of answer choices that you have concluded are incorrect. Keep in mind, however, that there will be times when you will have not eliminated any answer choices. In these cases, it is still a good idea to write the question number down along the left hand column, as you may use it in answer choice elimination at a future time.

When you have gone through all of the questions for a particular section, it is a simple task to jump to the questions that are unanswered or marked. However, minimize leaving any unanswered questions, "just in case."

Another tip is to make use of the computer "hot keys." For example, you may use your mouse to click on a particular choice or menu command. Instead of using the mouse, which takes a few seconds to maneuver over the item you wish to click, use the keyboard counterparts, which will appear as underlined text. By saving a few seconds for each question, you will cumulatively save minutes on the exam (*Note: this tip will not work for many of you, so use your judgment*). However, don't try this on the reading comprehension section since the mouse helps you scroll up and down the computer screen smoothly. It also serves as a convenient tool to help you keep your place while reading the text.

Yet another simple trick to save time is to avoid looking up at the amount of remaining time. During your planning and practice for this exam, determine a set of intervals that you will look up at the clock. Pertaining to the Survey of Natural Sciences section, one example would include, looking up at the 10th question, the 30th question, and further 20 question intervals. The first check will help you to know what kind of pace you have set. It is early enough that changing the pace will have a noticeable effect on the overall speed that you have set for that particular section. Also, it is delayed enough, so that you won't be prematurely altering what may have otherwise been a good pace.

Speed	Very slow pace	Slow pace	Ideal
Remaining at 5 minutes	20-30 questions	10-15 questions	0-5 questions
Strategy	Guess on all moderate and difficult questions. Answer only those questions that are easy or very short.	Guess on all difficult questions, but mark these problems. Answer all easy and moderate questions. If time permits, revisit the marked questions.	You're doing great! Just make sure that you are not missing too many questions during your practice exams when answering questions at this pace.

Table 4. Three general scenarios. All scenarios are based on the number of questions remaining with 5 minutes left on a 100 question exam. You may view these as percentages of questions remaining, and correlate them with various sections of the DAT.

A "mandatory" check should occur at about 5 minutes remaining, and another one at 1 minute remaining. The rationale for this is that at 5 minutes, depending on how much of the exam remains to be completed, you can begin to institute your "emergency" plan. Consider the scenarios listed in *Table 4*. In the first example, at 5 minutes you may still have a third of the exam left. While this should most certainly be outside of any original plans, you must have a backup plan. If you are in this situation, you should begin by guessing (often without reading the questions or answer choices) on all of the difficult questions. Pause only long enough to give you a *feel* of the difficultly level of a particular question. If it is *easy*, then take the time to answer it. If it is even remotely difficult, or if the question would take too long to read, just guess and move on. Your ultimate

goal is to fill in every single blank on the test, while picking out and answering the easy questions, thus minimizing your damages. It is worth losing a few hard questions that will eat up all of your time, in order to get to, and answer easy questions that otherwise would have been neglected. While it is unfortunate that anyone would ever find themselves in this situation, it happens all the time. Too often, a person under these circumstances will panic at their dire situation, and will continue at either a frantic pace, or even worse, will become paralyzed in their decision making abilities. This results in a horde of unanswered questions remaining when time is up.

The second and third scenarios are what is most likely going to happen for those students who have prepared themselves. In the second scenario, there are 15 questions left at the 5 minute check. At this point, it is very possible to finish right on time. However, there are doubtless a few questions that you left unanswered prior to this point. Thus, the wisest strategy would be to guess and skip the more difficult questions (make sure to make a mark on your grid for the ones that you guess on), and to spend some time answering the less difficult questions. The third scenario is an ideal one. This is the goal of proper time management. Remember, that rushing is counter-productive, and that proper time management is all about setting a good initial pace.

Always keep in mind the fact that the computer is unforgiving. Unlike a human proctor, who might look the other way as you are filling in your last circle, the computer will just shut off. Thus, at the 1 minute check point, make sure to fill in all of the blanks. DO NOT spend any time trying to solve any problems that remain. You will be sorely disappointed when the computer shuts you down. The only exception to this rule is if you find yourself with only one or two questions and you still have one minute left. Even then, just remember that a blank response is far worse than an uneducated one.

Proper Guessing

While not enough can be said about proper time management, an even less understood concept related to standardized tests is that of good guessing. Good guessing goes beyond simple deduction, elimination, and going with your hunches. It requires that you have some understanding of the guiding principle behind being *guaranteed* a higher test score. Granted, this guarantee is somewhat akin to a casino being guaranteed of ultimately making a profit off of every bet. Sometimes they pay money out, but the more common picture is of dealers raking money in. Similarly, there will be times that your guessing will result in less than anticipated numbers, and times when you will be lucky and score much better than you had hoped. In most cases, good guessing will result in numbers that live up to statistical expectations.

Consider the following situation. Peter and Mary are both taking the IT (Imaginary Test), an exam that is made up of 100 multiple choice questions with four answer choices, and to be completed in 50 minutes. First of all, tests like this, where there is barely enough time to read the questions and all of the answer choices, let alone to think about them, are written with the expectation that few test takers will complete them. The analogs in the DAT would be the reading comprehension, quantitative reasoning, and the perceptual abilities tests.

Continuing with the illustration, let's say that Peter and Mary are equally knowledgeable in the subject matter, and can be expected to answer all questions correctly when given enough time to complete the exam. However, both Peter and Mary are slow readers, and can only answer questions correctly at a rate of one question per minute. The only difference between these two test takers, is that Mary, being the wiser of the two, thought that instead of answering the last question, she would use that last minute to guess on the remaining 51 questions. So, Peter left the test having correctly answered 50 of the 100 questions. Mary left the test with a guaranteed 49 correct responses, but she had also completed the exam. That gives Mary a chance to receive credit on 51 questions. We all know, however, that it is almost impossible to guess correctly on 51 questions, especially if we haven't even seen the question (this would be similar to winning the lottery, so please don't rely on luck to bring you through!). Conversely, we also know that it is rather difficult to miss all 51 questions, even if we haven't had a chance to see them.

The statistical expectation would be a simple mathematical calculation of 51 questions divided by 4 answer choices per question. Thus, the result would be 12.75 correct responses. Mary's expected score, then, would be 62 out of 100. This is because 12.75 would, in most instances, round up to 13, and because she had read and correctly answered 49 other questions. On the PAT portion of the DAT, Peter's 50% correct score would probably result in a 15, whereas Mary's 62% correct score would most likely result in a 17.

In the above scenario, the additional 12% in score was achieved purely through blind guessing. In other words, just by finishing an exam, you will have a statistical advantage over the person next to you who leaves even one blank. An even more important lesson, is that there is an increase in your chances of correctly guessing, after you have made some deductions in the answer choices. That is another reason why, it behooves you to make a grid to keep track of the answer choices you have eliminated as possibilities, as was mentioned in the section on time management. Otherwise, you will have to reorient yourself with the answer choices, and this is unpractical.

While it is possible to achieve stellar scores with the combined implementation of good guessing with good deduction abilities, it is always better to rely on proper time management skills. This is because, reading a question in its entirety, will enable you to forego wasting time on answer choices once you have found the correct one. This saves you time in the long run. Also, you will have the best odds of answering a question correctly only if you have read the question. Also, to properly utilize your deduction skills, you will have had to have read the question, again pointing to the importance of proper time management.. Remember that guessing, while an important tool, is more or less, a gamble.

To see common standard score and raw score equivalents used in the DAT, as well as common DAT averages and percentile conversions, see *Appendix B* and *Appendix C.* You can look up your new target goal, and find out how many questions you need to answer correctly to achieve it. Also, you can estimate the percentile ranking that you will have if and when you achieve your target DAT scores. This is a simple way of estimating how many questions that you can miss for each section of the exam and still come out with the final scores that you want.

Other Advice

There are other things that you can do to increase your overall score. The biggest concept that is neglected by almost all DAT takers, is that of averages. While the score for the PAT portion of the exam is based solely on your performance on that section, the academic average of the DAT is an average of five sections. Too many students believe that scoring high on the basic sciences will guarantee them a high score on the DAT. First of all, remember that the scores reported by schools are the academic average and the perceptual ability scores. Although it would ideal to score high on the sciences, this may not always be achievable. Also, even if you score high on the sciences, but attain a mediocre score on reading comprehension and quantitative reasoning, your academic average will drop like a rock.

Because the academic average is made up of five scores, the sciences will only have a 3/5 weight on the final average. The other 2/5 is made up of reading comprehension and quantitative reasoning. Let's say that you score 20's for each of your sciences. On the other two sections you score 15's. Your overall score would then be [(20x3)+(15x2)]/5, or an average of 18. That's a drop of 2 points, which is huge in terms of percentile rankings! According to *Appendix C*, this drop of 2 points in the academic average translates to a fall of over 11 percentile points. Therefore, a wise person would try their best to inflate their reading comprehension and quantitative reasoning scores. To be honest, these two subjects cover areas that *every* college graduate should know and be proficient in. Consider the opposite example. Let's say that instead of 15', you score 22's (very high scores, but definitely attainable in these sections of the exam). Your new average would be 21! Yet a more common example would be as follows. Let's say that one of your science scores suffers for one reason or another. So you have a 20, 20, 15, 22, and 22. The average for these is a very respectable score of 20.

Finally, here are section specific hints and tips that may help some of you. The advice will differ from section to section.

For the **survey of natural sciences,** follow the detailed information at the beginning of this chapter concerning the purchase of a strong MCAT review book, and the specific areas of inquiry to become familiar with. Knowing the material, strengthening your weaker subject areas, and guessing after a thorough round of deduction will net the highest scores. Time is usually not the enemy here. Rather, a lack of knowledge, or indecision are the common problems.

There are three reading passages in the **reading comprehension** section of the DAT. You are given 50 minutes to answer approximately 15 questions for each of three reading passage (the actual number of questions will vary depending on the test and the reading passages). This section is a boon for those who have good reading skills, and a curse to those who abhor anything that has to do with reading. To add to the latter group's discomfort, you have to read quickly, just to finish this section. The key here is time management. Set a quick pace starting with the first reading selection. By the time you arrive at the third reading selection, you should have 15 to 20 minutes remaining. The best thing to do is to purchase a SAT review book from our list of recommended titles. These review books will provide you with a large amount of resources for both this section and for the quantitative reasoning section. Be sure to time yourself with the time limits that will be on the DAT.

When you are taking the test, you may want to jot down on your scratch paper, keywords or something to help you remember what that passage was about. For slower readers, try skimming. To do this, you will want to read the first paragraph of the passage, perhaps the second paragraph, all of the thesis sentences of the supporting paragraphs, and all of the conclusion paragraph. By doing this, you will know where to look to find detailed information for specific questions. Also, you will have a firm grasp of what the passage is about, what the author's feelings are concerning the subject, and other less objective topics. While practicing for the exam, think about constructing a mental "map" of the passage. Remember, that all of this information will be purely short term. Therefore, you should answer all of the questions pertaining to a passage before moving on to the next one. Otherwise, you might as well just guess, since remembering everything from a previous passage is very difficult.

Some of you may be tempted to go straight to the questions. Because the passages for the DAT are based mostly on detail type questions (the questions will usually ask specific details from the reading passage), this method may seem to work. However, you will waste a lot of time searching through the information, and you may become lost or fatigued. Keep in mind that the reading passages are not on paper. The computer screen can only hold so much information, and more often than not, if you go "searching" blindly for answers to questions as mentioned here, you will be swamped. Also, you will have no clue as to how the author felt about the subject, what attitude the passage reflected, etc.

When you reach the 5 minute check point (a personal check point as mentioned above in the *Time Management* section), be sure to have your back up plan ready. If you have many questions left, blindly guess on all of the lengthy questions (i.e., What attitude did the author feel towards the migratory trends of Canadian geese during the time period of 1985-1992?). These type of questions take a little over a minute to adequately read the question, the answer choices, and to think about a correct response. On the other hand, answers to simple detail type questions (i.e., What year were these migratory trends detected?), are much easier to find in the passages, especially if you've got a "map" of the passage in your mind. Remember, as with all sections, at one minute, just make sure to fill in all of the blanks.

The best way to study for the **quantitative reasoning** portion of the DAT, is to purchase a SAT book from our recommended list of review books. The only information that you will be lacking is the trigonometry portion of the DAT version of the exam. To study for the trigonometry, refer to an old text book, or browse through an ACT review book at a local bookstore. There are very few questions on trigonometry, and of the ones that are asked, they are usually very basic. Thus, purchasing a trigonometry review book may be a waste of time and money.

Go through the SAT review book in a systematic fashion. Make sure that you understand the concepts of a given topic before moving on to another one, as they are interrelated. As you begin to take practice math exams, start timing yourself as if you were taking the actual test on the DAT. Start to identify your weak points, and proceed to strengthen them. As the test date nears, and certain types of word problems are still causing you trouble, you should begin to think about them as a sacrifice. Sacrificing other types of problems is not advised. The two main benefits of sacrificing difficult word problems are: you will have a lot more time for the rest of the math problems, and you will feel a lot less anxious when you are faced with a difficult word problem. Be sure to keep the 5 minute checkpoint, and at 1 minute remember to fill in all of the blanks, including questions you may have skipped without having entered a guess.

The PAT

The **perceptual ability** portion of the DAT is probably the least understood part of the exam. It is also the only truly unique portion of the DAT exam, and is an important indicator to admissions committees of your ability to "see" things the way a dentist is required to see them. While the PAT is not the strongest indicator of clinical success in dental school, it does cover principles and concepts that will be utilized on a daily basis in dental school, and more importantly, in the real world. You will encounter problems that require the ability to interpret two-dimensional and three-dimensional figures. Often, this requires some mastery of mental manipulation of objects that are represented as lines and drawings on a flat surface, i.e. the computer monitor. These skills represent to some degree, the test taker's potential ability to adequately interpret radiographs (x-ray films), to successfully orient themselves in the oral cavity, and to feel comfortable working in an environment that often involves limited visibility. While the PAT may not accurately reflect your own potential success in the field of dentistry, it is a simple was to "weed" out those applicants that may pose an unnecessary challenge or risk in their clinical roles of dentistry.

To master this part of the test, you must fully understand the rules. To begin with, the PAT is made up of 90 questions, and is to be completed in 60 minutes. There are six sections to the PAT, with each containing 15 questions. As you take the diagnostic exam provided by the ADA (this exam is the best practice exam currently available), you will find that there are some sections that are relatively simple, while others are extremely difficult. The reason for this is that the more difficult sections are counterintuitive, the rules are poorly understood, the goals are hard to visualize, and the pressure of being timed just compounds these factors.

Let's begin with a brief summary of what is expected of you on this portion of the examination. The PAT is comprised of the following six sections: keyhole/shadow problems, top view-front view-end view exercises, angle determination and ranking, hole punch exercises, multiple block/cube counting, and pattern folding problems. Each section consists of 15 questions, bringing the total number of questions to 90. With only 60 minutes given for the exam, each question will have an average of 40 seconds available to it. If you are not already familiar with the PAT, you will soon learn that there are "easy" sections, and there are "hard" sections. In a test situation, you will find that the actual amount of time spent on easier problem types will be very small, while the harder problems will take up most or all of your remaining time.

The greatest increase in your score will come from being acquainted with the rules of each exercise. You must read and familiarize yourself with the rules that are listed for each section of the PAT. The exact rules are listed in the PAT portion of the sample DAT that is included with the DAT application materials. We have provided short summaries of the rules, as well as some detailed explanations and tips that might help you to shave a few precious seconds off of each question you may encounter. Please note, that while the test makers have designated each of the 6 sets of exercises as parts 1 through 6, some liberty has been taken of providing my own names for these individual parts. You will not see these names on the actual examination. Instead, you will see the part numbers assigned with each set of rules. Your ultimate goal is to skip the instructions and rules screens on the computerized PAT, as they are the same rules that are listed here. This alone will save you a large amount of time that would otherwise have been wasted.

Part/1
Keyhole or **shadow** exercises:

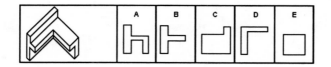

(The correct answer is C. The object is inserted through the opening with its left side entering first.)

1. *The object can enter the openings from any orientation, even from one that is not directly visible.*

Meaning-If you can imagine any object in three-dimensions, you will find that it has six basic sides to it: left, right, front, back, top, and bottom. Rule 1 is saying that this object can be inserted into one of the possible openings in any of those 6 orientations.

Tip-Instead of openings, or keyholes, think of shadows. If you shine a flashlight on a three-dimensional object, you will always get a two-dimensional projection. You can try this by shining a light on any object of your choice. Try to imagine the shadow that will be projected before you actually see it. This simple exercise will help you note small details that you may have overlooked. By thinking in terms of projections, you can narrow the possible orientations down to just three: right, front, and top. To find the other 3 orientations, simply "flip" the projection over. That is, imagine the mirror image of the projection. This mirrored image is the projection of the opposite side of the object! For example, if you were to flip a right side projection, you would be looking at the projection of the object's left side. This is a tremendously useful skill, as you can shave a significant amount of time from these problems by enhancing your level of deduction. If you find an opening that fits the mirror image of any of the object's projections, that answer choice is still the right answer! This is because, the mirror image, as mentioned above, is merely the projection of the other side of the object. If one of the answer choices fits the mirror image of the right side projection of the object, then the object will fit through the opening when inserted from the object's left side.

2.   *The object cannot be rotated once it has begun passing through the opening. The object's external outline it always the same shape as the correct opening.*

Meaning-Think about a circle and a square of the same diameter and length of a side, respectively. It is obvious that the circle can easily fit through the square. However, this is "not allowed." The projection of the object must be the exact same shape as the opening represented by one of the answer choices. The correct answer will not have spaces that remain unoccupied by the object as it passes through the opening.

Tip-Just make sure the answer choice fits one of the object's projections perfectly.

3.   *Objects and openings are drawn to the same scale. Therefore, the opening may be too small for the object, even though the shape of the opening may seem to be correct. Any differences in scale will be readily visible.*

Meaning-The opening must fit one of the object's projections like a glove. Not too big, not too small, but just right. There will be obvious differences in scale if two answer choices have the same shape, but are drawn to different sizes. The correct answer choice will be the one that is drawn to the same scale as the object.

Tip-Not too many questions will have answer choices that involve differences only in scale. If you encounter one, just pick the one that is closest in size to the correct projection of the object.

4. *There are no hidden irregularities in parts of the object that are not visible. Symmetry is preserved when it is implied.*

Meaning-What you see is what you get! The parts of the object that are hidden from your view, that is, the back of the object as well as part of its sides, will not contain any irregularities. You will always be given enough information to adequately answer each question. From that information, you will, at times, be required to extrapolate certain details. For example, when a straight line, flat surface, or other type of pattern is implied in the drawing of the object, it will be there. However, be careful that you are accurately interpreting the drawing and not just seeing things that are not being insinuated.

Tip-Keep in mind that this rule is different from the one in Part/5, block counting, where what you don't see, is not there, unless needed for support (more on this later).

5. *There is only one correct answer.*

Meaning-Only one answer choice is correct.

Tip-If you see mirror images within the answer choices, you automatically know that both are wrong. This is a quick and easy way to help whittle down your answer choices, as well as to double check yourself. If you just can't seem to "see" the projections in your head, try the following exercise. For each of the keyhole questions that you've finished, draw each of three projections on a sheet of paper: Top projection, Side projection, and Front projection. Remember that only the external outline of the object is important in each of these projections for this section. As you begin this exercise, you may not see the "correct" answer in your drawings. This may be due to several factors. First, your drawing may not be to scale. Second, you may have missed important details in drawing the projections. Third, you may be forgetting that the mirror image of a given projection also qualifies as the correct answer. The rationale for this is that the object can be turned around 180° to produce the reciprocal projection. Thus, the mirror image of the correct answer is also the correct answer.

Part/2
Top View-Front View-End View exercises:

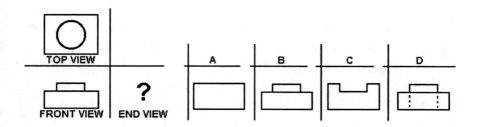

(The correct answer is B. Only B presents an accurate "view" from the object's right side. The top view may suggest that B or C is correct, but the front view eliminates C as a possibility. Answer choice A lacks the necessary details shown in both the top and front views. D is incorrect as it implies line or angle changes that are deeper in the object as seen from the right side. If this were the case, the front view would also indicate dotted lines that would corroborate the implications of D.)

1. *The following diagrams present the top, front, and end views of various solid objects.*

Meaning-There are three views relevant to the object. These are the top view, the front view, and the end view, or the view of the right side of the object (see *Figure 3*). Also, the object is solid and three-dimensional, having no hidden compartments, unless such compartments are implied in any pertinent views. So, if there is a hollow cavity in the object, you will know by the insinuations drawn in one or more views of the object.

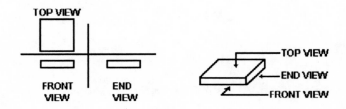

Tip -When you think about the three views, think of yourself as a helicopter pilot viewing a massive three-dimensional structure. Approach the object from above, looking down on the top of it. Next fly down to the front of the object noting how the details from the top relate to those on the front. Then, maneuver to the right side of the object to finish your "fly-by." This will help you to better envision, in a three-dimensional sense, the two-dimensional drawings that are given.

2.   *All views are drawn without perspective*

Meaning-The various views are drawn so that you do not see a tapering effect on the far portion of the object. The best comparison would be to an architect's drawings or floor plans, which are also drawn without perspective. Once the building is built, however, the effect of perspective is readily evident. For example, when looking at the font of the building, you will see the sides of the building heading towards a center point somewhere off into the distance. Another example would be a long road. As you look further down the road, it will seem to narrow in the distance.

Tip-This rule never seems to be a problem until people start thinking about what perspective is, and why such a rule even exists. Just don't worry about perspective, since it's not even part of this exam!

3.   *The Top view is located in the upper left hand corner of a cross, and is analogous to looking down on the object. The Front view is located in the lower left corner of a cross. The End view is located in the lower right corner of a cross. All views are labeled and are always in the same relative location for each question.*

Meaning-This rule is pretty self-explanatory. The important point here is that the views are analogous to looking at the object from each viewpoint. That is, looking down on the top of the object, looking forward at the front of the object, and looking sideways at the right end of the object. Also, the orientation of the three views relative to a cross, will be consistent from question to question, and will also be labeled. For each question, one of the three views will be missing, and will be denoted with a question mark. This is the view that you are expected to extrapolate from the two other views which will be given.

Tip-Remember that you are a helicopter pilot observing this large object from three separate vantage points. Always keep in mind that there may be hidden lines and angles, which will be represented as dotted lines. These hidden features may be solid lines in a different view if they can be seen directly, or they may be seen as dotted lines in a different view if there are line or angle changes that cannot be directly seen, but are in fact submerged beneath a given surface of the object.

4.   *Lines that cannot be seen directly, are represented as dotted lines.*

Meaning-If a line, or angle change is hidden behind a wall or surface, then it will be drawn as a dotted line (see *Figure 4*). By inference, any directly visible line or angle change is depicted as a solid line. Keep in mind that what may be a dotted line from one viewpoint may very well be a solid line from another view. Sometimes, a solid line will continue as a dotted line, both visible from one view. If this is the case, part of the line or angle change is directly visible, and part of it is not.

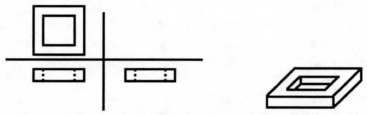

Figure 4. Top, front, and end views of a three-dimensional object. Remember that the views will always be presented in this fashion relative to a cross: the top view will be located in the upper left corner, the front view will be in the lower left corner, and the end view will be found in the lower right corner. Note how the solid lines in the center of the object from the top view are depicted as dotted lines in both the front and the end views.

Tip-This concept is not so easily demonstrated through words, but imagine looking at an easy chair from the front (*Figure 5*). There will be many solid lines, as there are many angle changes in the curvature of the chair frame and arms. From the side (*Figure 6*), however, the seat of the chair is hidden behind one of the arms of the easy chair. Therefore, the seat portion would be depicted as a dotted line from the end view, since the seat is there, as evidenced from the front view. However, from the end view, its presence is merely blocked from direct visual contact, due to the high arms of the easy chair.

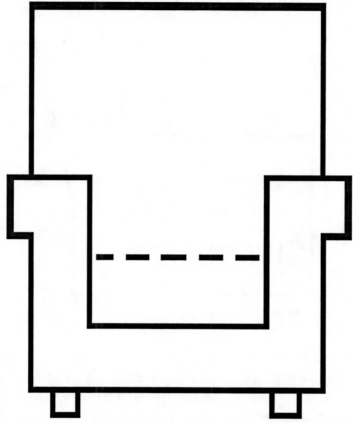

Figure 5. *Front view of an easy chair. Pay close attention to the arms, seat, and the back of the chair.*

There are a few other details to note. From the front view, the dotted line represents the angle change of the back of the chair as seen from the end view. Notice how the legs of the chair are the same in both views. This is because each of the legs is identical in shape, and there are four of them, two in front and two in back. Besides the seat being depicted as a dotted line, the back of the seat is also dotted where it drops below the level of the chair's arms. Don't forget that *any* angle changes are also considered as lines. Thus, an angle change that is directly visible will appear as a solid line. An angle change that is hidden by a surface will be drawn as a dotted line.

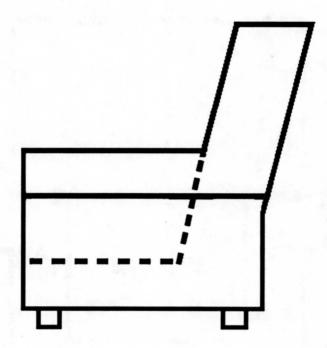

In addition, looking at the arms of the chair as seen in the front view, are seen as a solid line from the end view of the chair. An important thing to notice is that the level of the lines, whether solid or dotted, coincide with other lines and angle changes on the exact same levels, in this case, from top to bottom. That is, the lines for the arms are drawn in the end view at the same level (from the top of the chair to the bottom of the chair) that they are drawn in the front view. Similarly, the dotted line in the front view is drawn at the same level (from top to bottom) as it is in the end view (where it is represented as an angle change in the back part of the chair). For practice, try drawing the top view of the chair. Try to incorporate every detail shown in both the front and end views. Conceptually, think of the unknown view in terms of the six fundamental directions: top and bottom, front and back, left and right. This is one of the most important ideas related to this section of the PAT. By practicing these problems, you will gain a firm grasp on the interrelationships of these six directions and the three views. *Table 5* summarizes these relationships. Familiarity with this information will help you to mentally picture the object and the unknown view.

	Top View	**Front View**	**End View**
Top View		Left to Right	Front to Back
Front View	Left to Right		Top to Bottom
End View	Front to Back	Top to Bottom	

Table 5. Directional interrelationships between the top, front, and end views.

Part/3
Angle Determination and Ranking exercises:

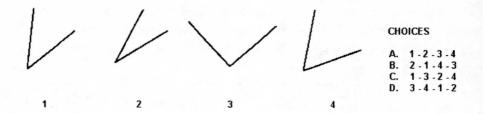

CHOICES

A. 1 - 2 - 3 - 4
B. 2 - 1 - 4 - 3
C. 1 - 3 - 2 - 4
D. 3 - 4 - 1 - 2

(The correct answer is B.)

1. *These angles represent interior angles.*

Meaning-All angles will be less than 180°.

Tip-Just make sure not to take too much time on this section. Experienced test takers have all demonstrated that trying to evaluate angles that are really close only eats away at the time, and usually doesn't help much in making a final determination. Instead of wrestling with angles that are close calls, go with your first instinct, and don't second guess it unless it later appears to be way off.

2. *Rank the angles from small to large.*

Meaning-Of the four angles that are drawn on the screen, correctly rank the angles from least to greatest in terms of degrees. Just think "small to large."

Tip-The "best" way to approach angles is to first locate the smallest and the largest angles. Next, eliminate incorrect arrangements from the answer choices. Usually, this will get rid of at least one answer choice, but every once in awhile, you may not eliminate any possible choices. You will often find that the answer almost presents itself once you've eliminated the incorrect possibilities. After narrowing down the choices, you will most likely find yourself having to decide between two angles: the two smallest, the middle two angles, or the largest two angles. Usually, the difference is readily detectable, but sometimes it is really difficult to tell the difference between two angles. In this case, go with your initial gut instinct and move on, noting the question number on your grid. If you have any time left over, come back to that question and try to answer it as soon as you see it. This way, you will be using your gut instinct to help you along.

Part/4
Hole Punch exercises:

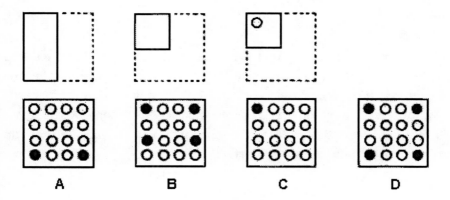

(The correct answer is D. The paper has been folded twice. Thus, it is four layers thick.. After being unfolded, the hole punch in the upper left corner has been mirrored on two planes–the same planes in which the paper was originally folded.)

1. *A flat, square piece of paper is folded one or more times. Broken lines indicate the original position of the paper, and solid lines indicate the position of the folded paper. The folded paper never leaves the original boundaries. The paper is never turned or twisted.*

Meaning-Basically, this rule is stating that each problem begins with a flat, square piece of paper. This piece of paper can be folded one or more times. For every fold, a dotted line will appear, which represents the previous position of the paper. For example, for the first fold, the dotted line would represent the original position of the square, flat piece of paper. Along with the dotted lines, there will also be solid lines, which represent the new position of the folded paper. These solid lines are usually visible in a direction away from the dotted lines, as the paper is folded away from the dotted lines. The paper always remains within the original square space, never leaving the space even during a fold. The paper is not twisted or otherwise bent in any way other than the simple folds insinuated by the dotted and solid lines.

Tip-Always be aware of previous folds. Sometimes, it is difficult to determine the direction in which a fold was made. Forgetting even one fold will result in an incorrect answer. The test makers, counting on this common error, have answer choices that seem to corroborate these faulty conclusions. Be careful and take your time, making sure that you get as many of these questions correct!

2. *There are 1 to 3 folds per question.*

Meaning-There will be at least one fold, and no more than 3 folds for any given question.

Tip-You should proceed to answer the single and double fold questions quickly and easily. Just be careful not to rush too fast. For the triple fold questions, take your time. A little extra time spent to guarantee a correct answer is well worth it for this section. Also, remember that every time a sheet is folded in half, the total number of layers rises by a factor of 2. For example, a sheet that is folded 3 times will have a total of 8 layers. The first fold creates 2 layers, the second fold makes 4 layers, and the third fold doubles that to 8 layers. For the first fold, where you have two layers, a single punch would create two holes. For the second fold, where you have four layers, a single punch would make 4 holes. And for the third complete fold, which would have eight layers, a single punch would result in 8 holes. Remember, there can only be a maximum of sixteen holes, as there is no space on the paper for anymore than that. Also, be careful to look out for folds that may seem to have this doubling effect, but do not since they are not completely folded in half. Rather, they may have a total layer count of 3, 5, 6 or 7 layers in some areas of the folded paper, and 2, 4, and 8 layers in other parts of the paper. This may result in an interesting final number of holes. For these questions, the number of total holes cannot be determined just by knowing how many layers are present. This is because the punch on these questions might be on just one layer, two layers, three layers, and so forth. So, you have to keep track of how many layers were punched in each question to be able to accurately predict the total number of holes.

You may be wondering why this concept is even mentioned here in such depth. By accurately predicting the total number of holes in a particular question, you can "double check" your answers to some degree. For example, if you chose an answer choice that shows eight holes, but by counting the layers you know that there will only be six holes, you will be able to correct yourself. Also, you can use this technique of predicting the number of holes to help you to eliminate answer choices that fall outside of your predictions. While this technique might seem lengthy, with practice it will quickly become second nature to you. With proper implementation, you should only be adding a few seconds to the time it normally takes you to answer each question. At the same time, you will be providing yourself with some added security. Remember to be careful since this is one of the easier sections!

3. *When the last fold is made, a hole is punched in the paper. After the hole is punched, mentally unfold the paper and decide on the final position(s) of the hole(s) on the original flat sheet.*

Meaning-After all the folding is done (1, 2, or 3 folds per question), a hole is punched in a portion of the folded paper. It is your job to mentally unfold the paper back to its original flat, square position, and determine where the holes will be located on it.

Tip-This all sounds a lot harder than it really is. If you're having problems visualizing it, try folding square sheets of paper for yourself (square Post-it® notes are great for this), then use a hole puncher to simulate the diagrams in this section of the PAT. Upon unfolding the paper, you will find the correct pattern depicted on the unfolded sheet of paper. This is an excellent way to practice for this section. Keep in mind that on the actual DAT, it has been reported that more than one hole may be punched. This makes the unfolding process much more complex. As mentioned before, try using prediction techniques, and please be careful! Finally, a white hole on the *final folded* sheet represents the area where a hole is punched. On the answer choices, which represent the unfolded sheet, areas of the paper that remain intact will be seen as white circles. Also, black circles represent the final pattern of punched holes once the sheet of paper has been unfolded back to its original shape and position.

Part/5
Block or Cube Counting exercises:

In Figure Z how many cubes have two of their exposed sides painted?

A. 1 cube
B. 2 cubes
C. 3 cubes
D. 4 cubes
E. 5 cubes

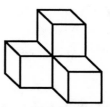

Figure Z

(The correct answer is A. Both of the two cubes seen on the bottom have four of their sides painted. The top cube has five of its sides painted. The *invisible* cube, the one supporting the top cube, will have two of its sides painted.)

1. *Each group of questions will be based on a figure made up of cubes of exactly the same size which have been cemented together. After cementation, the cubes are painted on all exposed surfaces. This includes the back and side surfaces, which are not directly visible. Only the bottom surface of the cubes remains unpainted.*

Meaning-For this section, you will be presented with several groups of problems each based on a given figure. This figure is composed of blocks or cubes which have been arranged in various configurations. They are subsequently cemented together on all the cube surfaces which come in contact with other cube surfaces. In the sample question above, this would mean a total of three cemented surfaces. After cementation, the group of cubes is painted on all *exposed* surfaces. This includes the surfaces on the back and side, both of which are not directly visible. Besides the surfaces which have been glued together, the only universal surface that is not painted is the bottom surfaces of the cubes. The reason for this is that the cubes are resting on a surface. So, when they are painted, this bottom surface cannot be reached, and are left untouched. An example of this is spray painting an object. After resting the object on a flat surface, you proceed to spray all exposed surfaces. All joints that have been glued, in addition to the entire bottom surface of the object, will remain unpainted.

Tip-At first glance, cube counting seems rather simple. Be careful though, not to fall for misleading visual "information" given in each figure. There are common pitfalls which you should avoid. First of all, know which types of cubes make up the various categories of cubes with painted surfaces. That is, know the various situations in which one, two, three, four, and five surface cubes can appear. Note that there is no cube that has six surfaces painted, although a cube is by definition made up of six sides. Also, know that there are cubes that may have none of their sides painted. These cubes are usually found at the bottom of a stack, and are surrounded on all sides by other cubes. Finally, remember that a surface must come into complete contact with another in order to avoid being painted. Thus, diagonal contact would still necessitate paint on any surface which would still be visible. Visibility includes direct visibility, which involves surfaces that are apparent in the figure (top, front, and the surfaces of one side), and indirect visibility, which involves surfaces that would be visible if you could physically rotate the group of cubes into direct vision (surfaces of the back and the other side that is not directly visible).

2. *There are no hidden cubes, except for those that are needed to pro-vide support for other cubes which can be seen.*

Meaning-What you see is what you get, sort of. While this rule might seem similar to Rule 4 of the Part/1 Keyhole or Shadow exercises, the exception given to cubes needed for support makes it significantly different. Think about the skyline of a big city. You will see tall skyscrapers in the background, and in front, you will see shorter buildings. Does this mean that the skyscrapers are just hanging in mid-air behind these shorter buildings? Of course not! The same logic applies to this rule. There are cubes that cannot be seen because they are either blocked out on one or more sides, or because they are on the other side of the figure. There may also be cubes that are totally hidden from any view. These cubes are implied and necessary to the overall configuration of the figure as they may provide the foundation for cubes placed above them, which are ones that we can see. So, if you can't see it, it's not there. Unlike the Keyhole or Shadow rule, symmetry is not implied in cube counting questions.

Tip-This concept takes some practice to master. At first, you may not see all of the cubes, and your answers always seem to come up short of the correct one. There are several ways to overcome this. The first is through knowing how to identify how many, and what type of cubes are present. You may try to use building blocks (which can be found in a children's toy store) to help visualize the figure by reconstructing it. Then carefully count how many cubes make up your reconstruction, as well as, what "type" of cubes they are. That is, count how many surfaces are exposed for each cube, and note it on a piece of paper. This will strengthen your visual perception of the "flat" figures on the real exam. Another technique to use after you have gained a firm grasp at visualizing every single cube, is to write numbers on each visible cube denoting the number of surfaces that are exposed on the cube. Do this for each cube. This includes ones that are obstructed from direct view, including all supporting cubes. Draw arrows in the general direction of the cube to help you keep track of which number goes with which cube. Next proceed to the questions and just tally up the numbers of cubes that are present in the figure. While this method used to be encouraged on the written DAT, you will not be able to use it on the computerized exam, unless you want to make marks on the computer screen. Use this method purely as a tool to help you practice, to build up your speed, and slowly wean yourself from writing the numbers physically to counting them in your head. If you are weak in this section, you will be surprised at how quickly you will excel after using the suggestions mentioned here.

Part/6
Pattern Folding exercises:

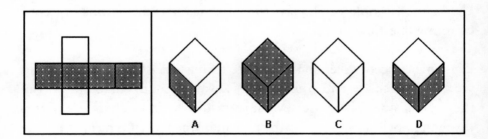

(The correct answer is D. It is important to note that while all answer choices are capable of matching the shape of the pattern on the left when it is folded, only D exhibits the proper shade configuration.)

1. *For questions in this section, a flat pattern will be presented. You are to fold each pattern into its proper three-dimensional form. There is only one correct answer for each question.*

Meaning-For pattern folding questions, you will be given a flat pattern on the left side of each problem. On each pattern you will see solid lines, which mean that the pattern is to be folded along each line. After making each fold, you should mentally arrive at a three-dimensional figure that corresponds to one of the answer choices on the right. There is only one correct answer.

Tip-Pattern folding tends to be one of the more difficult sections for most test takers. There are several reasons for this. First, the interpretation from two to three dimensions often results in a mental image that may not appear similar to any of the answer choices. Second, when various shading patterns are included, test takers will often choose the reverse answer. That is, they will choose the mirror image of the correct answer. Third, some of the questions are just plain hard. For these questions, a good practice exercise is to draw each flat pattern on a blank sheet of paper, but to a much larger scale, making sure to accurately represent the proportions, shading patterns, and all solid lines. Next, cut the pattern out following its external outline. Finally, fold the pattern along the solid lines, and you will see a three-dimensional object begin to emerge. With clear tape, make sure that the object is stable in its final shape. Now rotate the object to simulate the angulation presented by your answer choices. You should find that one of the answer choices matches the proper configuration and shading of your folded object. When you do this exercise, pay close attention to what it is that you are doing. Each step, from folding to rotating, has a mental counterpart. These physical steps that you take will ultimately need to be translated into mental manipulation skills for the real test. For some questions, you should be able to arrive at the correct answer quickly. These questions will involve unique shapes in the flat pattern itself. To capitalize on this, just look for the same unique shape in the answer choices. Once you find it, mentally double check your answer by quickly folding the flat pattern around the unique shape. Remember that there can only be one correct answer. As with the keyhole or shadow section, if you find two answer choices that are merely different perspectives of the same folded pattern, then both of those choices are incorrect. This is especially pertinent when the proper shading configuration of a pattern is the only item being tested.

2. *In each pattern presented on the left, you are looking at the outside of that pattern.*

Meaning-For each question, the flat pattern shown on the left side of the problem represents the outer surface of the final folded object.

Tip-Many test takers do poorly in this section because they fold the pattern towards themselves, or "out of the page." While in most cases this might result in the correct shape of the folded object, it will cause the shading pattern of the object to be backwards. That is, by folding the object towards yourself, you will end up with the mirror image of the correct pattern configuration. The test makers have set plenty of traps to exploit this common error. To arrive at the correct answer you must fold the pattern "into the page," or away from you. By doing this, you should mentally be looking at the bottom, or base, of the object, as opposed to looking at the top of the object, which would be the case if you had folded the pattern in the other direction. Next, you should mentally rotate the folded object so that you are "looking" at it from the same angulation as the one presented in the answer choices. The correct answer should be evident. Some test takers just cannot seem to fold the pattern away from themselves, or into the page, but have no problem folding the pattern in the other direction. If you find yourself in this situation, go ahead and continue folding the object towards yourself, or out of the page. However, when choosing an answer, you must reverse any shading patterns that you may be visualizing to arrive at the correct one. In other words, the correct answer will be the one that is the mirror image of the folded object that you are mentally visualizing. Whether you choose to fold the pattern "correctly" (away from yourself), or if you want to continue to fold the pattern towards yourself, just remember to be consistent with your folding methodology. Only through practice will you be able to achieve a level of consistency that will eliminate any doubt you may have when choosing your final answers.

Suggested Time Limits

As mentioned before, the key to succeeding in a test where time is the main constraint, is proper time management. This is especially true for the PAT. Having familiarized yourself with the PAT, you should now suspect that you will be spending a greater amount of time on some sections, and less of it on others. Rather than thinking in terms of an average amount of time per question for the entire PAT, try to allot your 60 minutes according to the various sections of the exam. In *Table 6* you will see a list of recommended times for each of the six sections of the PAT. These are only guidelines, and you should not hesitate to alter them to suit your particular needs. For example, if you need more time for hole punching, but are able to complete keyholes quickly, plan on shifting more minutes towards the weaker area. Once you have found a proper balance, stick with it, especially as your actual test date approaches. When taking the exam, it is advised that you only check your remaining time during the difficult sections. That way, you will not hamper your quicker pace for the easier sections, and you will be able to alter your slower pace for the more difficult sections. When time begins to run out, remember that all questions are worth the same. Therefore, guess and move on from the harder questions, and answer the easier ones.

	Recommended time per section	Recommended time per question	*Your* final pace
Keyholes	9 minutes	36 seconds	
Top View, Front View, End View	14 minutes	56 seconds	
Angles	4 minutes	16 seconds	
Hole Punching	5 minutes	20 seconds	
Cube Counting	9 minutes	36 seconds	
Pattern Folding	14 minutes	56 seconds	
Review/ Guessing	5 minutes	varies by number of unanswered questions	
Totals	60 minutes	40 seconds	

Table 6. Recommended times for the PAT. These are only guidelines that may vary from person to person. In the last column labeled Your final pace, enter the amount of time that you feel is needed for each section. Always try to reduce the time you need for each section.

5. What You Need to Do Today and Other Advice

The first thing you should do is make a time line. At the beginning should be the day that you plan on beginning your review process. Key points should be noted along the way to serve as reminders of important events that you should be preparing for, both mentally and emotionally. The reason for this is that many people don't realize the numerous steps and paperwork that will need to be completed somewhere in between planning to go to dental school, and actually getting that letter of acceptance. On the following page, you will find that *Table 4* has an example of important steps with corresponding blanks that you should fill in with important dates. Once you've finished this time line, the next thing you should do is follow it!

Before you proceed with the implementation of your time line, purchase a bound, lined notebook of some sort. This will be your DAT and dental school planning notebook, and will help you keep track of what you have done, what still needs to be done, contacts at various schools, notes from your review sessions, questions that you may have, and any other information that you may want to keep handy. This is the simplest method of organization for all of your DAT and dental school related thoughts and resources.

The first step is reviewing for the DAT. By now, you should have an idea of what method you wish to pursue. Hopefully, you are leaning towards the "do-it-yourself " method. If this is the case, go back and review chapters 3 and 4, paying close attention to the suggestions mentioned there. If you have chosen to take a test preparation course, then you should contact the test preparation center as soon as possible. Information on how to reach the more popular test preparation centers is available on the Pre-Dental Info web site, located at *www.predental-info.com*. Keep in mind that taking a test preparation course is rather expensive, so it would be wise to research which test prep course is best suited to your needs. For those of you who opt to look over old course notes, though this is discouraged, try to use some of the references and suggestions mentioned in this book.

While reviewing for the DAT is vital, you must make every attempt to ensure that your paperwork is submitted in a timely manner. This includes registering for the DAT as well as registering for the Associated American Dental School Application Service (AADSAS). The registration process for the DAT includes filling out an application form and submitting an application fee. An application form can be obtained by contacting the American Dental Association (ADA). Contact information for the ADA is available in Chapter 6. Registering for the AADSAS is a similar process. Simply contact the American Dental Education Association (ADEA) in order to receive an application form. You may also want to register online over the web at the ADEA website. Further contact information, as well as web addresses, can also be found in Chapter 6.

The Steps	Start Date	Finish Date
Review for the DAT		
Register for the DAT		
Choose your schools		
Submit applications through AADSAS		
Return secondary application	1) 2) 3) 4) 5)	1) 2) 3) 4) 5)
Interviews	1) 2) 3) 4) 5)	1) 2) 3) 4) 5)
Acceptance reply and deposit	1) 2) 3) 4) 5)	1) 2) 3) 4) 5)
Register with FAFSA		

Table 7. "Fill-in" chart for key steps in the dental application process. Copy this chart, fill it in, and post several copies in areas that you will see on a regular basis to remind you of your due dates.

Recently, the ADEA has dramatically increased their fees for processing the AADSAS. This is unfortunate, and smells very much of price gouging, since the ADEA has a virtual monopoly over pre-dental students regarding the dental school application process. This is especially true in light of the fact that many schools still require an additional application fee, and often a secondary, or supplemental, application form to be completed. The recent downturn in the number of dental school applicants compared to previous years may be partly to blame for this, and so may the decreasing number of post-graduate residency programs that are participating in the ADEA's post-doctoral application service. Nevertheless, submitting the AADSAS will be needed in order to be considered by most North American dental schools.

It is recommended that you carefully select 5 to 10 dental schools for serious consideration. After thoroughly investigating each of these programs, you should limit your selection to no more than five schools. Despite narrowing down your possible school choices, you may still wish to send your application to more than three schools. However, doing this will increase the overall cost of your application fee, currently at a cost of $40 for each additional school.

Use the suggestions, especially those found in Chapter 2, when making your final choices. Avoid the shotgun approach to applying to dental school. That is, don't send your application to every school available, or for that matter, to more than 10 schools. This is a total waste of money, in light of the fact that you will only be attending one of them. Applicants who "shotgun," usually have not carefully considered their career goals, and have not taken the time to investigate the resources that are readily available to them.

To begin with, you should choose one "dream" school (one that you would love to attend, but you're not exactly banking on being admitted into). At least three schools should be ones that you think you will be relatively competitive, in terms of being admitted, as compared to other applicants. Your final schools should be the one or two that you are almost positive that you will be admitted to. It will be up to you to make your final selection of three schools. It would be wise to consider *all* of the factors surrounding each program as you whittle down the possibilities. If you just can't seem to narrow down your search, you should reevaluate what it is that you are looking for in the dental school you wish to attend. If you have any questions regarding the application process for either the DAT or the AADSAS, please contact the ADA or the ADEA, respectively.

Registering Early for the DAT and the AADSAS

It is important to register for both the the DAT and the AADSAS as soon as possible. The reason for registering early for the DAT is obvious. By doing so, you will ensure yourself an opportunity to take the test on the date and at the location of your choice. The logic behind registering early for the AADSAS is somewhat more obscure. The benefits of early registration lie with the admissions process used by dental schools known as rolling admissions. Rolling admissions begins with the acceptance of applications, usually from the AADSAS application service. AADSAS generally begins accepting applications starting in June. The deadline for applications to participate in the AADSAS service depends on the specific deadline for each school.

Many people make the mistake of thinking that applying by the deadline is adequate. This is a deadly mistake in the rolling admissions process because most schools begin accepting applicants by the end of September to the beginning of November, although acceptance letters are usually begin to arrive by late November to early December. Often, more than half of the offers for a spot in the incoming class are made by the end of the year. Sadly, some people will wait until the application deadline to apply, a date set from September to March, with most schools setting their deadlines from January through March. For most of these schools, by the time the application deadline arrives, almost all of the entering class has already been selected. There may only be a few spots left open, and any remaining interviews are for those candidates who will probably be put onto a waiting list. It is common for candidates who are put onto a waiting list to never actually enroll for the year in which they are applying. This is especially true for candidates who are on the waiting lists of the more competitive institutions. Thus, it is essential that you submit all of your applications well in advance of any deadlines. Also, remember that the posted deadlines are not post mark dates, but are actual deadlines that the application must arrive to the ADEA. For more details, consult the AADSAS instruction booklet.

With rolling admissions, a candidate with average credentials who applies early, will have a better chance of being admitted into a particular program than a candidate with high marks who applies close to the deadlines. In fact, even borderline applicants will have a good chance of having their applications looked at by an admissions committee if they have their applications in early. The reason for this is that a school must fill up its entering class.

If you look at the ratio of accepted applicants to matriculated or enrolled students, you will find that generally speaking, that ratio will be about two to one. The reason for this is that every school is aware of the fact that one candidate may be accepted to more than one school. A person may "sit on" an acceptance offer from a school, by either waiting until the last possible moment before rejecting an acceptance offer, or be merely sending in the admissions deposit, which will reserve a spot for them in the incoming class. While this is usually a significant amount of money, students tend to ultimately go to their first choice school.

Often, an applicant will be accepted early by one program, and won't want to lose that spot for any number of reasons. At the same time, he or she would like to wait for more programs to respond. Sometimes, an applicant is placed on a waiting list for their top choice school, while being accepted to a school of lesser choice. In this case, the applicant will secure their spot at the latter school by paying the enrollment deposit, and will wait. In some cases, they will even wait for the entire summer of the year that they will be entering dental school. If they make it from the wait list of their top choice school to acceptance into the incoming class, they will, in effect, alter the original class roster for the school where they have secured a spot. In the process, they will forfeit any deposit monies paid to hold their place in the school they no longer plan to attend.

Keep in mind, the biggest reason that schools enroll more than they can handle is that many students who are accepted will reject a particular school's offer in favor of another school. In some cases, a student may have changed their career plans, or may wish to delay their entrance into dental school due to some unforseen circumstance. Dental schools, in an attempt to avoid having to scramble to fill their rosters at any point in the future, will accept roughly twice the number of students as there are spots in the program. *This may not be true for the specific program that you are applying to.* This information can be attained by asking the school how many people they accept, and how many spots they will have for the incoming class. While this ratio changes from school to school, and from year to year, it is always a rule to "over book" an incoming class. The moral of all of this is to APPLY EARLY!

The AADSAS Essay

Applying to dental school can be a daunting task. In addition to choosing the schools where your application will be sent to, you will be asked to answer numerous questions regarding your personal information, and you will be responsible for transferring your entire post-secondary educational history onto the application form. One word of advice when filling out the AADSAS, and any standardized form for that matter is to always err on the side that benefits you. If you have any doubts regarding *exactly* what the application is asking for, always interpret the question or the information request in your favor. Don't fabricate work experience or meritorious efforts, but it won't hurt to let your life accomplishments shine, and to elaborate on any particular item when the opportunity presents itself.

The AADSAS will also require an essay to be included with the rest of the application materials. If you can recall your high school days, when you were in the midst of applying to a post-secondary institution, you probably won't remember much about the torment you may have suffered while trying to concoct a witty, saintly, or otherwise intelligent essay. That's because, when you stop to think about it, the essay was, for lack of a better word, a formality. This does not mean that you can skip the AADSAS essay, nor does it mean that you can just write a flaky description of your summer watching Dr. XYZ pulling wisdom teeth all day. A strong essay may determine the fate of a "borderline" applicant. For example, if there are two applicants and only one spot remaining, the essay may become one of the deciding factors in determining which one is accepted.

The essay is also an opportunity for you to accomplish one or more of the following things, which are listed in order of importance: 1) an opportunity for you to explain a matter not adequately covered by the rest of the application that can be used to your benefit, 2) an opportunity to present meritorious and scholarly achievements that have brought you to this point in your life, 3) an opportunity to demonstrate your command of the English language, 4) an opportunity to elaborate on any volunteer activities that influenced your decision to become a dentist, and 5) an opportunity to wax eloquent on how and why you want to become a dentist. Some of these opportunities are specifically given through specific questions in the application form. However, by tying your awards, leadership positions, work experiences, or volunteering efforts into the essay, you will produce an essay that is unique, interesting, and will ultimately positively affect your application. Let's review each of these opportunities, starting from the least important.

Opportunity #5: You may be wondering why the story behind your decision to become a dentist is at the end. While it is important to comment on the factors influencing your decision to become a dentist, the reason that it is not of prime importance is that *every* applicant will write the same sort of thing. This may include stories of how the applicant decided to become a dentist due to their home town dentist, who was active in the community. Or, how their "familiarity" with the dental chair (as a frequent patient) piqued their interest in the field. Or, how their parent or relative is a dentist and just loves their profession. The list goes on and on.

Opportunity #4: The key to including a powerful reason as to why you want to become a dentist, is to involve other factors that do not center around you. This can include a description regarding any mission work (in any health care field) that you may have been involved in, or of the volunteering that you did at a local hospital or community dental clinic, or how you were an active participant (or even better, the organizer) of some local charity work, or even how you spent a summer helping out in a big brother or big sister program.

Opportunity #3: Communication skills are key to every aspect of life. The field of dentistry is no exception. By writing a well thought out, well organized essay, you will automatically separate yourself from the rest of the applications. A strong command of the English language is something that every graduate school looks for in a candidate. In dental school, the obvious reasons for this include your ability to comprehend the didactic material, and your ability to communicate clearly with your professors, peers, and most importantly, your patients. Also, if you indicate that you have an interest in research or academia, your sentence construction, grammar, verbal skills, and the flow of your writing will present a glimpse into your ability to convey your thoughts and ideas.

Opportunity #2: If you have nothing in your academic or personal record to explain, then this is the most important opportunity. Even though there are specific questions in the application regarding leadership roles, awards, and other meritorious and scholarly achievements, the same principle applies here as in *opportunity #4*. That is, you must be able to make your achievements relevant to why you are applying to dental school. There is nothing that an admissions committee or an interviewer likes better, than to see a well rounded, academically qualified individual. By relating your accomplishments to your decision to become a dentist, your application will stick out like a sore thumb. Ideally, every applicant should be able to showcase their achievements, but in reality, with the exception of a few schools, this will not be the case..

Opportunity #1: For candidates who have something to explain, either in their academic or personal history, the most important element of the essay is the opportunity to make the admissions committee understand why such discrepancies exist. This does not mean that you have to advertise minor blips in your academic record, nor does it mean that you have to you have to make excuses for anything in your personal life. However, if this information is relevant to where you are today, and if it can convey a true sense of who you are, then including it will only help your cause. Although there will be specific questions allowing you to "explain yourself," it will only help your cause if you adequately account for problems in your grades, since these are, by far, the most significant factors in the admissions process. For example, a sudden drop in grades might be due to a death in the family, a serious injury, a bout of depression, a bad ending to a significant relationship, a poor choice of undergraduate major, a drastic restructuring of the department's faculty or requirements, taking a job to pay for school, or just plain not knowing what you wanted to do with your life. Whatever the reason, however large or small it may be, don't be afraid to be honest about it. Believe it or not, admissions committees are made up of human beings, who can sympathize, and often, empathize with your particular situation.

Issues surrounding your personal history may include obstacles you have had to overcome, such as, a physical disability or a learning disorder. Family background issues may also be relevant, such as being the first in your family to attend college, or growing up in foster care. Whatever the issue may be, the fact that you have made it this far is a testament of your perseverance and willingness to succeed, even in the face of adversity.

When writing your essay, try to be concise. , and make sure that you proofread your final draft for any spelling, grammatical, or punctuation errors. Also, avoid hand writing the essay on the application form. Either type directly onto the form, or write the essay on a word processor using a type 10 font. Then, print, trim, and paste or tape (with invisible tape) the essay onto the application form. Make sure that the essay does not exceed the margins of the essay space on the application form. The black border of the application form should remain visible. Try to keep the entire application as neat as possible, since first impressions are important.

Regardless of how witty or emotionally moving your essay turns out to be, remember that this part of the application is much less important that your grades and your test scores. The good news is that most applicants with a GPA above 3.0 and/or a strong showing on the DAT's, as described in Chapter 3, will be accepted to a dental school, often the one of their choice.

Letters of Recommendation

Unless you have a really good reason not to, or unless you do not have access to one, you should have the pre-professional committee of your undergraduate school write a letter of recommendation for you. In virtually every instance, this recommendation letter will be positive.

A good reason to seek three individual letters of recommendation would be because you have access to three professors who know you personally, and who you know will write very strong letters of recommendation, in a timely manner, on your behalf. Also, if you have done any research, either independently or with a professor who is willing to write a positive recommendation for you, then you should consider this option. Even if a professor does not know you on a personal level, you may ask them to write you a letter of recommendation. However, prior to asking them to write a recommendation for you, be sure to ask them if they are willing to write a *positive* one. This can be done politely, and it is not rude to ask if the letter of recommendation will be positive. If the professor is not willing to write a letter of recommendation for you, this is usually a sign that any letter they may write will be a poor or negative one.

The Interview

Assuming that all of your application materials are completed and submitted in a timely manner, including any secondary or supplemental application forms, you can expect to start hearing from the schools. This process will begin to happen in the months of November and December and will usually continue until the end of March. You will be notified with one of two types of letters. The first type is a rejection letter. Do not feel discouraged if the first letter you receive is one of these. Even the strongest applicants will be rejected by one or more schools. There are many factors that come into play, such as in-state/out-of-state status, alumni connections, and the strength of the rest of the applicant pool for any given year.

The second type of letter is an interview letter. This letter will ask for you to call the admissions office to schedule an interview. There will usually be two or three dates that are available for you to choose from. If you receive more than one interview offer, try to schedule them so that you can interview at more than one program during a single trip. This may not always be possible, but some schools are willing to accommodate certain applicants who may have to travel a long distance to attend the interview, by allowing a privately scheduled interview session. If for some reason, none of the available dates will work for you, you may be able to schedule a phone interview.

Only schedule an interview at schools where you have a strong desire to attend, or schools that you feel confident of being accepted to. It is a waste of travel expenses and your time to interview at schools that you do not have a real interest in. However, interviewing at a school that you are relatively sure of being accepted into, is in your best interest. By doing so, you will feel more confident at future interviews by knowing what to expect during an interview, and by knowing, that in a worst case scenario, you have a school that you can fall back on.

Try to arrive at the interview site early enough to figure out how to travel from your hotel to the school itself without getting lost. Also, be sure to go to bed early, so that you will be well rested in the morning. Appropriate dress consists of a suit, or dress pants, along with a dress shirt and necktie, for men, and a suit, dress, or other business or semiformal wear, for women. Leave from your hotel room early enough to arrive at the school fifteen minutes early.

When you arrive at the interview session, you will most likely participate in an all-day program with many students. Refreshments and a lunch are provided at most schools. The day will usually begin with listening to a couple of introductory speakers, such as the dean of the dental school, the assistant dean for academic affairs, and the administrator who is in charge of the admissions process. After that, you will break up into smaller groups for a tour of the school's facilities, which is usually led by a dental student, followed by a personal interview. The order in which you participate in each scheduled activity will be prearranged. If you need to leave by a certain time, or cannot attend the morning portion of the program, make sure to inform the school ahead of time. In most cases, they will be more than happy to accommodate your needs, and will personalize your schedule accordingly.

During the tour of the school, you should ask any specific questions regarding the facilities, the patient pool, the requirements, and the tour guide's own opinion of the dental program. Avoid inundating the tour guide with too many detailed questions, since you will have an opportunity to receive an official response during your interview. If you really want the "lowdown" on a program, ask the tour guide if he or she is willing to give you their e-mail address. You will probably receive a more honest and detailed response this way.

When it is your turn to interview, according to the schedule, prepare yourself prior to seeing the interviewer. Visit the restroom and look in the mirror to reassure yourself that you are presentable. Before you go into the interviewer's office, take a deep breath and try to relax. Greet the interviewer by his or her proper title, maintain good eye contact during the introductions, smile, and shake their hand firmly. When you seat yourself, do not fidget, or change your seat position too regularly. Also, you may cross our legs, but do not cross your arms. Speak deliberately and calmly, answering each question with a firm and even voice.

You will be asked several "meat and potato" questions. These include: Did you have a nice trip? Did you find the school without any problems? Why do you want to be a dentist? Why did you choose this particular program? Can you elaborate on your experience in Dr. Smith's office? Would you describe your experience at the Hope Dental Clinic? Do you have any questions for me? If you have a blip on your undergraduate transcript, or on a specific section score of the DAT, they will also give you the opportunity to offer an explanation. However, if they don't bring up any of your academic shortcomings, do not bring it up yourself.

The types of questions that you will want to ask the interviewer include the following: When do students start seeing patients in the clinic, and in what capacity? What is the format of the clinic (comprehensive care versus quantity based)? What are the housing options and prices in the area? What sorts of transportation to and from the school should you be expecting? What types of research opportunities exist for you? How many students pass the national and state or regional boards? How is class ranking determined? What type of instruments will you be responsible for, or do they have an instrument loan program? Which basic science classes can you test out of? Do not ask the interviewer about the attrition rate, or about which residency programs exist at the school (unless they have a program that is truly unique), or about how many students get accepted. You should already know these answers prior to the interview. Most of this information is readily available in *The ADEA Official Guide to Dental Schools*. Information on how to order this book can be found in the next chapter. You can also find this information on the school's web site, or by calling or e-mailing the admissions office prior to the interview.

If you have a question regarding information that you feel would be important, don't hesitate to ask it. Hopefully, you will have written down all of your potential interview questions in your notebook, and attempted to find the answers on your own, well in advance of the interview. Also, before you leave for your interview, you should take another look at any questions that remain, and ask yourself if you really need to know the answers to them.

The whole point of this advice it to help you to present yourself as an informed, confident applicant. You want to use praises sparingly, but you never want to embarrass the interviewer with potentially negative questions. Always remember that as an interviewee, you have already passed the major hurdles for acceptance into the program, and for all practical purposes, you are accepted. The only person who can ruin it for you, is you.

The interviewer already knows that you are adequately qualified for the program, or you would not have been offered an interview. What they are looking for is strong communication skills, confidence, prior familiarity with the dental school, and general information regarding their program. They are also trying to make a determination about what type of person you are. Are you the type of person who will maintain the school's reputation? Do you exude a professional attitude? Are you courteous and respectful? Are you a mature individual? Are you prepared for the interview? These are aspects of a person's character that cannot be gleaned from an application form alone, and must be determined through a face to face meeting.

When you are finished with your interview, politely shake the interviewer's hand, smile, and say something to the effect of, "Thank you for your time, and for the opportunity to visit the school." The interviewer might dismiss you with a parting comment, such as, "It was a pleasure speaking with you, and I hope your trip back home is safe. You will be hearing from us in a few weeks or so.*

Other Advice...

When you receive an acceptance offer from a school, try to delay responding to it until one full week before the due date. This way, you can wait for other schools to make you an offer. As long as you send in the acceptance deposit before the due date, your place in the incoming class is assured. If you wish to reject an offer, notify the school as soon as possible, so that they can make an offer to another student. Also, send them a letter expressing your gratitude for their consideration of you.

If you accept an offer, start looking for a place to live immediately. You can correspond with current students for their opinions by requesting contact information from the admissions office. Also, while you were in the city during the interview, you should have picked up the local rental guide. This will give you an idea of what the housing market is like for the area you plan to live in. You can also browse the local rental and real estate market on the web. To get the most out of your money, however, you should look in the classified sections of the student and local newspapers. You can request the admissions office to send you a copy, or to provide you with the information on how to obtain one.

If you are wait-listed, this is usually a sign that you applied too late. If this is the case, you may be accepted sometime before the actual enrollment date. If you are ultimately not accepted into the incoming class, there is a strong likelihood that you will have no problem being accepted into the next year's class. Make sure that you are in regular contact with the school regarding your position on the wait list. Another reason that you may be put on a wait list, is that your application is "borderline" for the given year. Be sure to accept another school's offer, just in case you do not make it off of the wait list and into the incoming class.

When you receive the financial aid packet from the school, complete and return it as soon as possible. In most cases, you will be required to fill out the Free Application for Federal Student Aid (FAFSA_) form. This application can also be completed on their web site (www.fafsa.ed.gov). Send this form in by the school's requested deadline, even if you do not have all of the tax information on hand. You can always provide that information to the school's financial aid officer at a later date. Keep in mind, that to be considered for grants, you will most likely have to submit a copy of your parent's income tax return, in addition to your own. If you have specific questions regarding this process, or how to fill out the financial aid forms, contact the school's financial aid officer immediately. If you send the documents in too late, you may delay, or even lose, certain channels of money.

If you were not given one during the interview, you should request a book list of first year textbooks. The best way to determine which books to buy and which books to avoid, is to contact a current dental student. They will be more than happy to share their experiences and information with you. Please do the same, and share your personal pre-dental experiences and useful information with others.

6. Additional Resources

In this chapter, you will find valuable information regarding organizations, references, and other dental related resources. With the increasing popularity of the Internet, most of these organizations have their own web sites, where you can find out more information about them. Also, often times, they will provide easy avenues of communication via e-mail. This is a great way to quickly get the information that you need straight from the source. Since this book is not affiliated with any of these organizations, information regarding them may change without any notice. *Disclaimer: neither the author nor the publisher of this book has any financial or administrative interest in any of the organizations, publishing companies, or test preparation centers listed in this chapter.* For your convenience, you can find all of these resources, fast links to their web sites, along with newly updated information at the following web site:

http://www.predentalinfo.com

If you have any dental related questions, you can can ask them on the Pre-Dental Info mailing list. Information on how to subscribe is on the web site. If you have a special circumstance that you would like Dr. Kim to comment on, you can contact him via e-mail at: drkim@predental-info.com.

Dental Related Organizations and Resources

ASDA

To join the American Student Dental Association (ASDA) as a pre-dental member, use your web browser to go to:
http://www.asdanet.org/member/predental.htm

To find out more information about ASDA, go to:
http://www.asdanet.org

You can contact ASDA by writing to:

ASDA
211 East Chicago Avenue, Suite 1160
Chicago, Illinois 60611
Telephone: (312) 440-2795

ADEA

To receive an American Dental Education Association (ADEA) form for their application service (AADSAS) as mentioned in Chapter 5, or to apply online, point your web browser to:
http://www.adea.org/AADSAS/AADSAS_Main_Page.htm

or, send the following information to the address below: 1) your name, 2) a daytime telephone number, 3) your complete address, 4) the year in which you plan on entering dental school (i.e. "Entering Class of 2002"), and 5) a written request for the current AADSAS application. You may also call their toll-free number to request a copy.

ADEA
1625 Massachusetts Avenue, NW, Suite 600
Washington, DC 20036-2212
Telephone: (202) 667-9433
                (800) 353-2237

The ADEA also has other very useful publications. A full list can be seen at:
https://www.adea.org/publications/Order/orderform.htm

To receive the highly recommended publication *The ADEA Official Guide to Dental Schools* (formerly known as *Admission Requirements of U.S. and Canadian Dental Schools*), as mentioned in Chapter 5, send a $35 ($40 if outside the U.S. or Canada) check or money order payable to ADEA, or your Visa/MasterCard/American Express account information to:

ADEA
Attn: Publications
1625 Massachusetts Avenue, NW
Washington, DC 20036-2212

If you prefer, you can order using you VISA, MasterCard, or American Express over the phone by calling (800) 353-2237.

ADA
To register for the DAT, you'll need a DAT application from the American Dental Association. You can request this application at:
http://www.ada.org/prof/ed/forms/test-app.html
or, send the following information to the address below: 1) your name, 2) a daytime telephone number, 3) your complete address, 4) the year in which you plan on entering dental school (i.e. "Entering Class of

2002"), and 5) a written request for the current DAT application and preparation materials.

American Dental Association
211 E. Chicago Avenue
Chicago, Illinois 60611
Telephone: (312) 440-2500

You may also want to purchase their DAT Tutorial. While it does not cover any test material, it will help to familiarize you with the process of taking the DAT. This tutorial can be requested by writing a request and sending a $10 money order to:

DAT Tutorial
Department of Testing Services
211 East Chicago Avenue, Suite 1846
Chicago, Illinois 60611

Please note that it is not recommended to purchase this tutorial as it only gives you a cursory introduction to the computerized DAT. To receive a more authentic computerized DAT experience, please refer to the *Top Score Pro* software mentioned later in this chapter.

DAT Test Preparation Centers

Test preparation centers are good for test takers who either feel as if they need external "enforcement" of a game plan, and for those who just don't feel comfortable preparing on their own. Personally, I strongly advocate the self-study method, since this is the only method that I have ever used to prepare for every standardized examination that I have ever taken. *I know that it can work!* This is not to say the seeking the aid of a test prep center is bad. However, you should be well aware that even with their materials and instructors, it still comes down to you. You must read the assignments. You must do the homework. You must ask the relevant questions. I have taught the DAT at one of the major and probably largest test preparation center in this country. I have reached the following conclusion: *In terms of knowledge and information, there is nothing that a test preparation center offers that cannot be self-taught or learned from much less expensive means.* The cost of attending a test prep center can range from approximately $1000 to over $2500 for more personalized instruction. Regardless, you will be taught, in most instances, by students who are not much more knowledgeable than you are! Therefore, it would be wise to begin your preparation for the DAT well in advance, utilizing the resources that you have around you, including professors, teacher assistants, and your peers. Once you begin to set a pace, and start to internalize your motivation to succeed, you will be guaranteed to score higher with self-study than with any other method.

Please visit **www.predentalinfo.com** *for up-to-date information regarding DAT Test Preparation Centers.*

The following listings are current as of this book's publication date. However, if a more recent version of the titles are available, please don't hesitate to purchase the updated version. It may have additional resources, such as CD-ROMs, or may have information that has been corrected and updated.

For the most recent listings, please visit the Pre-Dental Info website at:

www.predentalinfo.com

Dental Related Publications-Recommended Titles

DAT Review Materials-Science Review

There are currently, several excellent science review books available for DAT test takers. While two of the texts recommended here are MCAT specific, the science review sections for each of them cover all of the major areas that you will be responsible for on the DAT. Take some time to visit your local bookstore and browse through these texts. By doing this, you will expose yourself to what is available, and you will be more likely to find a text that suits your individual style of review.

Of the few DAT specific review books that are on the market, only one adequately covers the basic science material that is going to be on the test. This book, *Kaplan DAT*, also includes reading comprehension and quantitative analysis questions, as well as a section on the PAT. Only the science section, however, seems solid enough to be considered for serious study for the DAT. It seems that Kaplan is merely publishing it's DAT prep course material in the form of a book. While they have some good points, the PAT section, for example, is fraught with errors, and are not adequately representative of the actual PAT section of the DAT. For this reason, it is not listed in the recommended list for study of the PAT, other than as a backup. *Avoid using any other DAT specific books in the course of your science review.*

Of these science review books, try to purchase only one, as the cumulative cost of review books begins to add up rather quickly, and the information between the different books is virtually identical. Remember, this is one of the few times that you will have to study as hard as possible. Once you have enrolled into a dental school, the experience of reviewing for the DAT will only be a fond memory.

Peterson's the Gold Standard MCAT: 2000-2001
2nd Edition

by Brett Ferdinand, Lisa Ferdinand, Kristin Finkenzeller

800 pages, February, 2000
Petersons Guides; ISBN: 0768901928; List Price: $44.95

Kaplan MCAT Comprehensive Review
Book with CD-ROM for Windows & Macintosh, 5th Edition

by Rochelle Rothstein (Editor)

1069 pages, October, 2000
Kaplan; ISBN: 0743201868; List Price: $65.00

Kaplan DAT
Book with CD-ROM for Windows & Macintosh

836 pages, October, 2000

Kaplan; ISBN: 074320185X; List Price: $55.00

For the latest science review books, and links to purchase them, visit *www.predentalinfo.com.*

DAT Review Materials-Reading Comprehension and Quantitative Reasoning

You may already be in possession of an earlier edition of one of these books. If you have a SAT review book, look through it before purchasing one at a bookstore. Reading comprehension tests, and the skills to do well on them have not changed appreciably to justify buying a new book if you already have one. The same logic applies to the quantitative reasoning section of the DAT. If you have an old SAT review book, make sure that it devotes sufficient attention to math problems, especially word problems, since this is usually the worst area for most test takers. The only way that you are going to increase your math skills, is to do as many different problems as you can. However, keep in mind that the DAT will cover some basic trigonometry, which is not covered in any SAT review books. This information can be found in an old math text book, or in an ACT review book. It is not advised to go out and buy a math review book just for the information on trigonometry, unless you feel like you are a little too rusty on math as a whole. If this is the case, plan on using a review book that covers all the aspects of the quantitative reasoning portion of the exam.

Barron's Sat I How to Prepare for the Sat I

21st Edition

by Sharon Weiner Green, Ira K. Wolf

824 pages, January, 2001
Barron's Educational Series; ISBN: 0764113909; List Price: $14.95

Sat & Psat 2001
Book with Cd-Rom Edition

608 pages, July, 2000
Kaplan; ISBN: 0684873346; List Price: $32.00

Remember, succeeding on both the reading comprehension and the quantitative reasoning sections demands practice! You must be comfortable with finishing the test sections with some time to spare. To begin with, avoid "hints" and other strategies. Turn to them only if your own techniques are not producing the results that you need to achieve the score that you want.

DAT Review Materials-Perceptual Abilities Test

As mentioned before, there is a true shortage of DAT preparation books. Fortunately, there are many other exams that cover materials that happen to overlap with most of the DAT. On the other hand, there are little to no review books that adequately cover the PAT portion of the DAT. Because the PAT is unique to the DAT, finding a strong review book is extremely difficult. Granted, there are several books out there, but none of them come close to adequately preparing the student to achieve their highest potential scores. As mentioned earlier, the Kaplan DAT book may function as a backup reference, but contains significant errors and deviations from what is to actually be expected on the real DAT examination.

However, there is one software title that we highly recommend. Although it does not give "tips," so to speak, it does provide an authentic computerized DAT experience.

TopScore Pro for the DAT, Computerized Sample Tests and Guide Version 7.0

by ScholarWare.com, Inc.

CD-ROM, September, 2000
ScholarWare; ISBN: 0967275709; List Price: $39.95

Dental School Admissions Information

The only written sources of information that you should use for dental school admissions planning are the materials published by the American Dental Education Association (see information listed earlier in this chapter). The reasons for this include: accuracy, up to date statistics, wide range of statistical categories, and other dental school related topics. You may want to check to see if your local library carries, or is willing to purchase, ADEA publications before spending your own money. If you find an older edition in your local library, don't despair. Statistics change very slowly from year to year, and in most cases, are otherwise accurate. Remember, your final source of dental school information should not come from a book. Rather, you should investigate each prospective school by speaking with current students and recent alumni, by requesting specific information from each school prior to applying, and finally, asking pertinent questions during your interview.

Dental Related Publications-Titles to AVOID

DAT Review Materials

The following is a list of titles that I have used, thoroughly reviewed, and just can't find a reason to recommend. If you want to check them out for yourself, please do so. Most of these titles are merely repackaged materials with little or no editorial changes for the past several years. Also, they provide no in depth review of basic sciences, reading comprehension, and quantitative reasoning skills. Of the little PAT review that may pop up in some of these titles, it is hard to justify spending your time reviewing with what amounts to be some rather inferior questions. You will be much better off with the practice exam that is found in the DAT registration and application packet, the practice exams found in the Top Score software package, and the soon to be released PAT specific review book, *The PAT Made Easy*, by Joseph S. Kim, DDS.

In the meantime, here are the list of books that I don't think you should purchase. However, I don't want to come across like I am putting down someone else's product. So, if you have the time, browse through them at your local bookstore, and draw your own conclusions.

Dat : Complete Preparation for the Dental Admission Test: The Science of Review

2001 Edition

by Aftab S. Hassan

256 pages, March 15, 2000
Lippincott, Williams & Wilkins; ISBN: 078172838X; List Price: $28.95

How to Prepare for the Dental Admission Test (DAT)

by Richard A. Lehman

496 pages, April, 1999
Barrons Educational Series; ISBN: 0764105779; List Price: $16.95

New Rudman's Questions and Answers on The...Dat : Dental Admission Test (ATS 12)

by Jack Rudman

April, 1999
National Learning Corporation; ISBN: 0837350123

and

Dental Admission Test

David M. Tarlow

January, 1993
National Learning Corporation; ISBN: 0837350123; List Price $23.95

(Note: these last two titles have the same ISBN number. Both are terribly poor review books and are not adequate for DAT preparation.)

Dental School Admissions Information

The reason for including the following book in the AVOID list, is that it draws the applicant's focus away from his or her true objectives. While this seems to be one of the "favorites" of statistics-minded pre-dental students, it is important to note that much of the information regarding the schools is inaccurate. Also, this book tends to make the reader want to apply to schools based solely on entering class averages, or other factors that should not be weighed so heavily. The information specific to dentistry is widely available from other sources, such as the ADA web site (www.ada.org). If you would just like something to look at to give you an idea of what the competition levels or tuition amounts are for dental schools in general, then this book fits the bill. If, however, you intend to use this book as your main book for admissions planning purposes, please leave it on the shelf, and look at it only in the bookstore.

The proper book for admissions planning is the ADEA publication, *The ADEA Official Guide to Dental Schools* . The reasons for this have been mentioned above, but deserve to be repeated. This guide, which is published on a yearly basis, takes the applicant information from the AADSAS applications filled out by each dental school candidate, and compiles it. Then, they publish pertinent information, such as DAT averages, GPA levels, number of applicants and number of enrollees, tuition costs, and much more detailed information. Even more importantly, these are official numbers that are published from the source. Another benefit of this publication is that it will give you information regarding who makes up the class (i.e., ethnic backgrounds, male and female, etc.), and also information regarding the school in general.

Barron's Guide to Medical and Dental Schools
Book with CD-ROM, 9th Edition

by Saul Wischnitzer, Edith Wischnitzer (Contributor)

624 pages, August, 2000
Barron's Educational Series; ISBN: 0764173758; List Price: $18.95

II.

Appendices

A. Schools and Addresses

Below is a list of dental schools in the United States and Canada. Also listed are the web addresses of the schools. Enter the entire web address into the address line of any web browser. This list is also available on the Pre-Dental Info web site at *www.predentalinfo.com,* along with direct links to each school.

This list is current as of the publication of this book. Current deans, associate deans, and other administrative persons may have changed. This should not present you with any problems, since in most cases, you will be communicating with the admissions office. When writing to a school, address your correspondence to "Admissions" or "Student Services." If you prefer to write an e-mail for more information, make sure it is directed towards one of these two areas. Most web sites will have links that you can click to automatically begin writing a letter. However, it may be wiser to just copy down the e-mail address, thus keeping the address on hand for follow-up purposes. There are also other technical issues that may also interfere with the smooth operation of directly writing an e-mail from a web site link.

Dental Schools in the United States

Alabama
University of Alabama School of Dentistry
1919 Seventh Avenue, S.Birmingham, AL 35294
Dr. Mary Lynne Capilouto, Dean
http://www.dental.uab.edu

California
Loma Linda University
School Of Dentistry
Loma Linda, CA 92350
Dr. Charles J. Goodacre, Dean
http://www.llu.edu/llu/dentistry

University of California at Los Angeles
School of Dentistry
10833 Leconte Ave., Rm. 53-038, CHS
Los Angeles, CA 90095-1668
Dr. No-Hee Park, Dean
http://www.dent.ucla.edu

University of Southern California
School of Dentistry, Rm 203
University Park-Mc 0641
Los Angeles, CA 90089-0641
Dr. Harold Slavkin, Dean
http://www.usc.edu/hsc/dental

University of California
School of Dentistry

513 Parnassus Ave., S-630
San Francisco, CA 94143
Dr. Charles Bertolami, Dean
http://www.ucsf.edu/campus/SchDen.html

University of the Pacific
School of Dentistry
2155 Webster Street
San Francisco, CA 94115
Dr. Arthur Dugoni, Dean
http://www.dental.uop.edu

Colorado
University of Colorado Medical Center
School of Dentistry
4200 East 9th Ave., Box C284
Denver, CO 80262
Dr. Howard M. Landesman, Dean
http://www.uchsc.edu/sd/sd

Connecticut
The University of Connecticut
School of Dental Medicine
263 Farmington Avenue
Farmington, CT 06032-5332
Dr. Peter J. Robinson, Dean
http://sdm.uchc.edu

District of Columbia
Howard University
College of Dentistry

600 "W" Street, N.W.
Washington, DC 20059
Dr. Charles Sanders, Dean
http://www.howard.edu/collegedentistry

Florida
Nova Southeastern University
College of Dental Medicine
3200 S. University Drive
Fort Lauderdale, FL 33328
Dr. Seymour Oliet, Dean
http://dental.nova.edu

University of Florida
College of Dentistry
P.O. Box 100405
Gainesville, FL 32610-0405
Dr. Frank A. Catalanotto, Dean
http://www.dental.ufl.edu

Georgia
Medical College of Georgia
School of Dentistry
1459 Laney Walker Blvd
Augusta, GA 30912-0200
Dr. David R. Myers, Dean
http://www.mcg.edu/SOD

Illinois
Southern Illinois University
School of Dent Med-Building
2800 College Avenue-Room 273/2300
Alton, IL 62002
Dr. Patrick Ferrillo, Jr., Dean
http://www.siue.edu/DMSCH

University of Illinois at Chicago
College of Dentistry
801 South Paulina Street
Chicago, IL 60612
Dr. Bruce S. Graham, Dean
http://dentistry.uic.edu

Indiana
Indiana University Medical Center
School of Dentistry
1121 West Michigan Street
Indianapolis, IN 46202
Dr. Lawrence I. Goldblatt, Dean
http://www.iusd.iupui.edu

Iowa
The University of Iowa
College of Dentistry
Dental Building
Iowa City, IA 52242
Dr. David Johnsen, Dean
http://dentistry.vh.org

Kentucky
University of Kentucky
College of Dentistry
800 Rose Street-Med. Ctr.
Lexington, KY 40536-0084
Dr. Leon A. Assael, Dean
http://www.mc.uky.edu/Dentistry

University of Louisville
School of Dentistry
Health Sciences Center
Louisville, KY 40202
Dr. John N. Williams, Dean
http://www.dental.louisville.edu/dental

Louisiana
Louisiana State University
School of Dentistry
1100 Florida Ave., Bldg. 101
New Orleans, LA 70119
Dr. Eric J. Hovland, Dean
http://www.lsusd.lsumc.edu

Maryland
University of Maryland
Baltimore Colegel of Dental Surgery
666 West Baltimore Street, Rm. 4-A-11
Baltimore, MD 21201
Dr. Richard R. Ranney, Dean
http://www.dental.umaryland.edu

Massachusetts
Boston University
Henry M. Goldman School of Dental Medicine
100 East Newton Street
Boston, MA 02118
Dr. Spencer N. Frankl, Dean
http://dentalschool.bu.edu

Harvard School of Dental Medicine
188 Longwood Avenue
Boston, MA 02115
Dr. R. Bruce Donoff, Dean
http://www.hsdm.med.harvard.edu

Tufts University
School of Dental Medicine
1 Kneeland Street
Boston, MA 02111
Dr. Lonnie H. Norris, Dean
http://www.tufts.edu/dental

Michigan
The University of Michigan
School of Dentistry
1234 Dental Building
Ann Arbor, MI 48109-1078
Dr. William E. Kotowicz, Dean
http://www.dent.umich.edu

University of Detroit Mercy
School of Dentistry
8200 W. Outer Drive

P.O. Box 98
Detroit, MI 48219-0900
Dr. H. Robert Steiman, Dean
http://www.udmercy.edu/htmls/dentistry/dental.htm

Minnesota
University of Minnesota
School of Dentistry
515 S.E. Delaware Street
Minneapolis, MN 55455
Dr. Peter Polverini, Dean
http://www.umn.edu/dental

Mississippi
The Univ of Mississippi
School of Dentistry-Medical Center
2500 North State Street
Jackson, MS 39216-4505
Dr. J. Perry Mcginnis, Dean
http://dentistry.umc.edu

Missouri
Univ of Missouri-Kansas City
School of Dentistry
650 East 25th Street
Kansas City, MO 64108
Dr. Michael J. Reed, Dean
http://www.umkc.edu/dentistry

Nebraska
Univ of Nebraska, Medical Center
College of Dentistry
40th & Holdrege Streets
Lincoln, NE 68583-0740
Dr. John Reinhardt, Dean
http://www.unmc.edu/dentistry

Creighton University
School of Dentistry
2500 California Street
Omaha, NE 68178
Dr. Wayne W. Barkmeier, Dean
http://cudental.creighton.edu

Nevada
University of Nevada
School of Dentistry
4505 Maryland Parkway, Box 453055
Las Vegas, Nevada 89154-3055
Dr. E. Steven Smith, Interim Dean
http://www.unlv.edu/dental_school

New Jersey
University of Medicine and Dentistry
New Jersey Dental School
110 Bergen Street
Newark, NJ 07103-2425Dr. Cecile Feldman, Dean
http://dentalschool.umdnj.edu

New York
State University of New York
School of Dental Medicine
325 Squire Hall
Buffalo, NY 14214
Dr. Russell J. Nisengard, Interim Dean
http://www.sdm.buffalo.edu

Columbia University
School of Dental and Oral Surgery
630 West 168th Street
New York, NY 10032
Dr. Allan J. Formicola, Dean
http://cpmcnet.columbia.edu/dept/dental

New York University
College of Dentistry
345 East 24th Street
New York, NY 10010
Dr. Michael C. Alfano, D.M.D., Dean
http://www.nyu.edu/Dental

State University of New York
School of Dental Medicine
Rockland Hall
Stony Brook, NY 11794-8700
Dr. Barry R. Rifkin, Dean
http://www.informatics.sunysb.edu/dental

North Carolina
University of North Carolina
School of Dentistry

104 Brauer Hall, 211 H
Chapel Hill, NC 27599-7450
Dr. John W. Stamm, Dean
http://www.dent.unc.edu

Ohio
Case Western Reserve University
School of Dentistry
2123 Abington Road
Cleveland, OH 44106
Dr. Jerold S. Goldberg, Dean
http://www.cwru.edu/dental/casewebsite

Ohio State University
College of Dentistry
305 West 12th Avenue
Columbus, OH 43210
Dr. Henry W. Fields, Jr., Dean
http://www.dent.ohio-state.edu

Oklahoma
University of Oklahoma
College of Dentistry
P.O. Box 26901
Oklahoma City, OK 73190
Dr. Stephen K. Young, Dean
http://dentistry.ouhsc.edu

Oregon
The Oregon Health Science University
School of Dentistry-Sam Jackson Pk

611 S.W. Campus Drive
Portland, OR 97201
Dr. Sharon P. Turner, Dean
http://www.ohsu.edu/sod/index.html

Pennsylvania
Temple University
School of Dentistry
3223 North Broad Street
Philadelphia, PA 19140
Dr. Martin F. Tansy, Dean
http://www.temple.edu/dentistry

University of Pennsylvania
School of Dental Medicine
4001 West Spruce Street
Philadelphia, PA 19104
Dr. Raymond Fonseca, Dean
http://www.dental.upenn.edu

University of Pittsburgh
School of Dental Medicine
3501 Terrace Street
Pittsburgh, PA 15261
Dr. Thomas Braun, Dean
http://www.dental.pitt.edu

Puerto Rico
University of Puerto Rico
School of Dentistry
P.O. Box 365067

San Juan, PR 00936-5067
Dr. Fernando Haddock, Dean
http://wwwrcm.upr.clu.edu/Dentistry.htm

South Carolina
Medical University of South Carolina
College of Dental Medicine
171 Ashley Avenue
Charleston, SC 29425
Dr. Richard De Champlain, Dean
http://www2.musc.edu/dentistry/dental.html

Tennessee
University of Tennessee
College of Dentistry
875 Union Avenue
Memphis, TN 38163
Dr. William F. Slagle, Dean
http://www.utmem.edu/dentistry

Meharry Medical College
School of Dentistry
1005 Dr. D.B. Todd Blvd.
Nashville, TN 37208
Dr. William B. Butler, Dean
http://www.mmc.edu/dent.htm

Texas
Texas A&M University System
Baylor College of Dentistry

3302 Gaston Avenue
Dallas, TX 75246
Dr. James Cole, Dean
http://www.tambcd.edu

The University of Texas
Health Sciences Center-Dental Branch
6516 John Freeman Avenue
Houston, TX 77030
Dr. Ronald Johnson, Dean
http://www.db.uth.tmc.edu

The University of Texas
Health Sciences Center-Dental School
7703 Floyd Curl Drive
San Antonio, TX 78284-7914
Dr. Kenneth L. Kalkwarf, Dea
http://www.dental.uthscsa.edu

Virginia
Virginia Commonwealth University
VCU-School of Dentistry
P.O. Box 980566
Richmond, VA 23298-0566
Dr. Ronald J. Hunt, Dean
http://www.dentistry.vcu.edu

Washington
University of Washington
School of Dentistry
Room D-322 Box 356365

Seattle, WA 98195
Dr. Paul B. Robertson, Dean
http://www.dental.washington.edu

West Virginia
West Virginia University
School of Dentistry
The Medical Center-P.O. Box 9400
Morgantown, WV 26506-9400
Dr. James J. Koelbl, Dean
http://www.hsc.wvu.edu/sod

Wisconsin
Marquette University
School of Dentistry
P.O. Box 1881
Milwaukee, WI 53201
Dr. William K. Lobb, Dean
http://www.marquette.edu/dentistry

Dental Schools in Canada

Alberta
University of Alberta
Faculty of Medicine and Oral Health Sciences
Room 3036 Dent/Pharma Bldg

Edmonton, Alberta T6G-2N8
Dr. G. Wayne Raborn,
Associate Dean For Dentistry
http://www.dent.ualberta.ca

British Columbia
University of British Columbia
Faculty of Dentistry
350-2194 Health Sciences Mall
Vancouver, B.C. V6T-1Z3
Dr. Edwin Yen, Dean
http://www.dentistry.ubc.ca

Manitoba
University of Manitoba
Faculty of Dentistry
780 Bannatyne Ave. Rm D113
Winnipeg, Manitoba R3E-0W2
Dr. Johann Devries, Dean
http://www.umanitoba.ca/faculties/dentistry

Nova Scotia
Dalhousie University
Faculty of Dentistry
5981 University Avenue
Halifax, Nova Scotia B3H-3J5
Dr. William A. Macinnis, Dean
http://www.dentistry.dal.ca

Ontario
University of Toronto
Faculty of Dentistry
124 Edward Street
Toronto, Ontario M5G-1G6
Dr. B.J. Sessle, Dean
http://www.utoronto.ca/dentistry

University of Western Ontario
Faculty of Medicine and Dentistry
1151 Richmond Street
London, Ontario N6A-5C1
Dr. Stan Kogon, Acting Director
http://dentistry.uwo.ca

Quebec
Ecole De Medecine Dentaire
Pavillon de Medecine Dentaire
Ste-Foy, Quebec G1K-7P4
Mme. Diane Lachapelle, Dean
http://www.ulaval.ca/fmd

McGill University
Faculty of Dentistry
3640 University Street
Montreal, Quebec H3A-2B2
Dr. James Lund, Dean
http://www.mcgill.ca/dentistry

Universite De Montreal
School of Dental Medicine
C.P. 6128 Succursale A

Montreal, Quebec H3C-3J7
Dr. Jean Turgeon, Doyen
http://www.medent.umontreal.ca/indexa.htm

Saskatchewan
University of Saskatchewan
College of Dentistry
107 Wiggins Road, Room B526
Saskatoon, Saskatchewan S7N-5E5
Dr. Charles G. Baker, Dean
http://www.usask.ca/dentistry

B. Common DAT Standard and Raw Score Equivalents

As with any standardized examination, the DAT implements a conversion from a "raw" score to a "standard" score. The raw score represents the actual number of correctly answered questions. The standard score is a number used by the testing agency to represent test takers' raw scores into something more practical and meaningful to the people involved in the admissions process. In the DAT for example, even though the number of questions may vary amongst subjects, they are represented along the same scale, that is, from 1 to 30. Thus, we hear of "scaled" scores, or in this case, a standard score. Note, that a range of raw scores may result in the same standard score. For example, under Biology, a raw score of 27-29 will result in a standard score of 17. That is, a score of 27, 28, and 29 will all result in a 17.

By itself, the standard score is meaningless. *The only thing that matters is how well you do relative to other test takers.* Therefore, the following tables should be used along with those found in *Appendix C*, in order to find out what these scores really mean. This can be accomplished by looking at the percentiles, since percentiles represent how well the test taker does relative to other test takers.

The following tables have been modified from a single table published by the American Dental Association. It is important to note that these conversions are only estimates of how your raw scores will be converted into standard scores for your particular examination. However, these tables can give the test taker a pretty good idea of where he or she stands amongst the rest of those taking the DAT, especially when used in conjunction with *Appendix C.* Also, note that the conversion for the reading comprehension section only shows 17 possible correct answers. This is because the conversion chart is based on the American Dental Association's practice examination materials. The actual reading comprehension section will contain approximately 50 items.

Standard Score	Quantitative Reasoning	Reading Comp.	Biology	General Chemistry
30	40	-	-	-
29	39	17	40	-
28	-	-	-	30
27	-	-	-	-
26	38	-	39	-
25	37	16	-	29
24	36	-	38	-
23	35	15	-	28
22	33-34	-	37	-
21	31-32	14	35-36	27
20	29-30	13	34	26
19	27-28	12	32-33	24-25
18	24-26	11	30-31	22-23
17	22-23	9-10	27-29	20-21
16	19-21	8	24-26	18-19
15	16-18	7	21-23	16-17
14	14-15	6	18-20	13-15
13	11-13	5	15-17	11-12

12	9-10	4	12-14	9-10
11	7-8	3	10-11	7-8
10	6	-	8-9	6
9	5	2	6-7	4-5
8	4	-	5	3
7	3	1	4	-
6	2	-	3	2
5	-	-	2	-
4	-	0	-	1
3	1	-	1	-
2	-	-	-	-
1	0	-	0	0

Standard Score	Organic Chemistry	Total Science	Perceptual Ability Test
30	30	100	90
29	-	99	89
28	29	98	88
27	-	97	-
26	-	96	87
25	28	95	85-86
24	-	94	84
23	27	92-93	81-83
22	-	89-91	78-80
21	26	86-88	74-77
20	25	81-85	70-73
19	23-24	76-80	65-69
18	21-22	70-75	59-64
17	19-20	63-69	52-58
16	17-18	56-62	46-51

15	15-16	48-55	39-45
14	13-14	41-47	32-38
13	11-12	33-40	26-31
12	8-10	27-32	21-25
11	7	21-26	17-20
10	5-6	17-20	13-16
9	4	13-16	10-12
8	3	10-12	7-9
7	-	7-9	6
6	2	5-6	4-5
5	-	4	3
4	1	3	2
3	-	2	-
2	-	-	-
1	0	0-1	0-1

C. Common DAT Standard Score and Percentile Equivalents

The following tables show the percentage of test takers who score equal to or lower than the standard score. For example, under the organic chemistry table, a standard score of 18 means that 82.4% of test takers achieve a standard score equal to or lower than 18. These numbers are published by the American Dental Association, and actual percentages may vary from year to year. Upon receiving your DAT scores, you will find that applicable tables will be published, usually on the reverse side of the score sheet that you will receive. Notice, that in almost every category, a standard score of 23 results in being in the 99th percentile (see *Appendix B* for information regarding raw score to standard score conversions). This translates to correctly answering roughly 90% of the questions for each section.

Quantitative Reasoning

Standard Score	Cumulative Percent
30	100.0
29	99.9

Reading Comprehension

Standard Score	Cumulative Percent
30	100.0
29	100.0

28	99.9	28	99.9
27	99.9	27	99.8
26	99.6	26	99.7
25	99.5	25	99.4
24	99.1	24	98.8
23	98.9	23	98.0
22	98.0	22	95.9
21	96.9	21	92.2
20	94.3	20	86.6
19	91.2	19	76.6
18	85.6	18	62.8
17	76.4	17	46.2
16	65.1	16	30.4
15	50.2	15	17.5
14	33.3	14	8.2
13	21.5	13	3.8
12	11.3	12	1.5
11	5.0	11	0.5
10	2.2	10	0.1
9	0.8	9	0.0
8	0.3	8	0.0
7	0.1	7	0.0
6	0.1	6	0.0
5	0.0	5	0.0
4	0.0	4	0.0
3	0.0	3	0.0
2	0.0	2	0.0
1	0.0	1	0.0

Biology		General Chemistry	
Standard Score	*Cumulative Percent*	*Standard Score*	*Cumulative Percent*
30	100.0	30	100.0
29	100.0	29	100.0
28	100.0	28	100.0
27	100.0	27	99.6
26	100.0	26	99.4
25	99.9	25	99.3
24	99.8	24	98.2
23	99.6	23	97.8
22	99.2	22	96.5
21	98.3	21	94.2
20	96.3	20	90.9
19	93.4	19	86.1
18	87.7	18	78.8
17	78.4	17	69.7
16	65.8	16	59.1
15	51.1	15	46.1
14	34.4	14	34.2
13	21.0	13	21.6
12	11.3	12	12.6
11	5.0	11	6.3
10	2.0	10	2.7
9	0.6	9	1.2
8	0.2	8	0.4
7	0.0	7	0.1
6	0.0	6	0.1
5	0.0	5	0.0
4	0.0	4	0.0

3	0.0	3	0.0
2	0.0	2	0.0
1	0.0	1	0.0

Organic Chemistry

Total Science

Standard Score	Cumulative Percent	Standard Score	Cumulative Percent
30	100.0	30	100.0
29	100.0	29	100.0
28	100.0	28	100.0
27	99.7	27	100.0
26	99.5	26	100.0
25	99.4	25	99.9
24	98.5	24	99.8
23	98.2	23	99.7
22	97.1	22	99.3
21	95.8	21	98.4
20	92.9	20	96.6
19	88.7	19	93.3
18	82.4	18	87.7
17	73.8	17	79.0
16	64.0	16	66.6
15	52.5	15	51.5
14	41.2	14	35.3
13	29.6	13	20.1
12	18.8	12	10.1
11	9.8	11	3.6
10	5.2	10	1.0
9	2.3	9	0.2

8	1.0	8	0.0
7	0.5	7	0.0
6	0.3	6	0.0
5	0.2	5	0.0
4	0.1	4	0.0
3	0.1	3	0.0
2	0.1	2	0.0
1	0.1	1	0.0

Academic Average

Perceptual Ability

Standard Score	Cumulative Percent	Standard Score	Cumulative Percent
30	100.0	30	100.0
29	100.0	29	100.0
28	100.0	28	100.0
27	100.0	27	99.9
26	100.0	26	99.9
25	100.0	25	99.8
24	99.9	24	99.7
23	99.7	23	99.4
22	99.3	22	98.5
21	98.3	21	97.0
20	96.2	20	94.1
19	92.3	19	89.3
18	85.4	18	82.9
17	74.0	17	73.4
16	58.6	16	60.9
15	41.1	15	46.4
14	24.3	14	31.1

13	11.9	13	19.0
12	4.6	12	9.1
11	1.3	11	3.8
10	0.3	10	1.2
9	0.0	9	0.3
8	0.0	8	0.1
7	0.0	7	0.0
6	0.0	6	0.0
5	0.0	5	0.0
4	0.0	4	0.0
3	0.0	3	0.0
2	0.0	2	0.0
1	0.0	1	0.0

About the Author

Dr. Joseph Kim is currently a resident at the University of Pittsburgh School of Dental Medicine. He received a Bachelor of Arts in Religion with a minor in Chemistry from Andrews University, located in Berrien Springs, Michigan, where he attended on a full Presidential scholarship. Dr. Kim received his Doctor of Dental Surgery degree from the University of Michigan in Ann Arbor.

Dr. Kim has consistently scored in the 99th percentile on all of his major high school and undergraduate standardized tests, including both sections of the DAT. He is a National Merit Finalist and Scholar, as preparation instructor for the PSAT, SAT, ACT, and DAT, helping students well as the recipient of numerous academic awards for scholarship. He has been a test understand the ins and outs of both the examinations as well as the admissions processes for undergraduate and dental education.

A husband and a father, Dr. Kim enjoys many hobbies in diverse fields. After completion of his residency training in Prosthodontics and implant surgery, he plans to enter private practice and to be associated with academic dentistry on a part-time basis.